SOS 4 TOTS

Tethered Oral Tissues™ • Tongue-Ties & Lip-Ties

*Exposing the myths about breastfeeding and healing
the heartbreak to make breastfeeding a joy*

LAWRENCE A. KOTLOW DDS

SOS 4 TOTS Tethered Oral Tissues™ • Tongue-Ties & Lip-Ties

For more information visit KIDDSTEETH.COM,
or contact the author, Dr. Lawrence Kotlow, via email: KIDDSTEETH@AOL.COM

Graphics: Jeff Radden
Animated Arts Schenectady NY 12203

Editor: Victoria Wright
Victoria@ BookmarkServices.net

Photos: Thank you Nash, Jessica, Jody, Josh, Caren, Lexie, Sophia, Emily, Andrew and Sharon

Book design by The Troy Book Makers
Printed in the United States of America
The Troy Book Makers • Troy, New York • thetroybookmakers.com

To order additional copies of this title,
contact your favorite local bookstore
or visit www.tbmbooks.com

ISBN: 978-1-61468-343-8

CONTENTS

LAWRENCE KOTLOW DDS

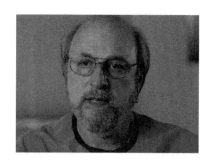

Dr. Lawrence Kotlow graduated from the SUNY Buffalo Dental School in 1972, and received his pediatric dental training as a resident at the Children's Hospital in Cincinnati, Ohio from 1972–1974. He established his dental practice in Albany, New York, in December of 1974. He achieved board certification in the specialty of pediatric dentistry in 1980 and is a fellow of the American Board of Pediatric Dentistry. Dr. Kotlow has received three prestigious awards from the State of New York Dental Association's Third District Dental Society, and he served as president of the Third District Dental Society and on many committees at the State level.

He is a member of the ADA, ICD, New York State Dental Association, Academy of Breastfeeding Medicine, American Academy of Physiological Medicine and Dentistry and the Academy of Laser Dentistry. As a member of the ALD, Dr. Kotlow served on its board of directors, achieved advanced proficiency in erbium lasers as well as standard proficiency in the use of diodes, CO_2 @9300nm and Nd: YAG lasers and ALD Mastership status. He was the 2014 recipient of the Leon Goldman Award for Excellence from the ALD. He has lectured on a wide range of clinical uses of lasers on infants and children, and establishing the ALD one-day pediatric program at the ALD annual session.

He is an internationally known expert on aiding mothers to achieve a comfortable and effective latch during breastfeeding with tongue-ties and lip-ties and has lectured to over five thousand health-care professionals on the diagnosis, laser treatment, and post-surgical care of these infants. He has lectured on lasers and pediatric dentistry throughout the United States and in Israel, Canada, Taiwan, France, England, Australia, and Italy.

He has contributed to textbook chapters on the use and benefits of soft-tissue lasers, hard-tissue lasers, endodontics and photobiomodulating lasers in pediatric dentistry in *Dental Clinics of North America 2004*, in *The Atlas of Laser Dentistry*, and in *Principles and Practice of Laser Dentistry, Lasers in Endodontics* . He has had articles published on laser dentistry in the *Academy of Laser Dentistry Journal, European Archives of Pediatric Dentistry, Journal of Human Lactation, Journal of Clinical Lactation, Journal of Orthodontics, Journal of General Dentistry, Journal of the Canadian Dental Association*, and many others.

He has been involved in the development and introduction of the isotopic carbon dioxide laser operating @ 9300nm known as Solea, developed and manufactured by Convergent Dental, a US company.

"As a parent who has had two children with tongue and lip ties, and as a clinician who has seen many patients struggling with the effects of both, it's been hard to find comprehensive, thorough and easy to understand information on tongue and lip ties. This book is an excellent resource for dentists, obstetrician-gynecologists, midwives, lactation consultants, pediatricians and parents who are looking for more information about how tongue/lip ties affect breastfeeding, speech, dental development and overall pediatric health. Dr. Kotlow has put it all into one convenient place!"

Heather Lane, CNM, MSN

INTRODUCTION

As a parent, you have great expectations for motherhood. Unfortunately for many mothers, breastfeeding becomes a toe-curling, painful experience because of poor or missed diagnoses of tethered oral tissues such as tongue-ties and lip-ties.

This book demystifies why, for some mothers, breastfeeding becomes a frustrating, painful journey, and for some infants, a miserable, painful beginning to life. I have been treating infants for breastfeeding difficulties due to tongue and upper lip-ties since 1974. In recent years with the increased number of mothers desiring to breastfeed their infants, I have revised over ten thousand abnormal frenum attachments of what are now referred to as "tethered oral tissues" (TOTs).

These TOTs are usually a combination of tongue-ties, medically known as ankyloglossia, and upper lip-ties. They require the release of the maxillary frenum and in some instances upper buccal and lower mandibular restrictive frenum attachments.

This book will dispel the myths concerning these TOTs, discuss the correct position in which to examine your infant to be able to correctly evaluate and find TOTs that are most often the cause of these symptoms and difficulties, and how to correctly and safely have these tissues revised.

If you are a mother who has been suffering needlessly, there may be times when you will cry as you read this book because you will realize the problems are not your fault; the professionals on whom you were depending for help had a basic lack of understanding. As a first-time mother, if you do develop problems, now you know to seek help before your symptoms overwhelm you.

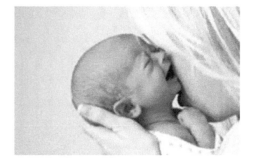

PART 1

Part 1 of this book is for mothers and fathers who have been searching for answers to why their infant has had a poor latch on the mother's breast, which has led to a significant number of problems for both the mother and infant.

It is a must-read for every mother desiring to breastfeed. It will also be informative to all health-care professionals.

CHAPTER 1

The Birth

For nine long months you have eagerly anticipated the birth of your child. The day finally arrives, and immediately after the baby is born, he or she is placed on your chest and the mother-infant bond begins.

You are relieved and excited. For months you have read about the wonders of motherhood and breast-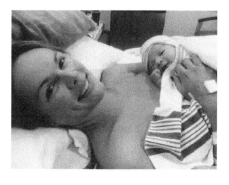
feeding and the lifetime bond that you alone can develop with your baby. As you lie there after a home birth or in the delivery area, your infant snuggles close and finds your breast, and the moment you have looked forward to begins. But something seems wrong. As your infant attempts to latch onto your breast, it hurts. You think, *Something is not right. This is not fun and enjoyable. What is wrong?*

For anxious mothers, this is a terrible introduction to motherhood. As the days go on and you are working to overcome your infant's inability to latch without causing you discomfort, all sorts of new symptoms begin to arrive. For you as the mother, your nipples may become raw, bleeding, flattened, and painful. Mastitis, plugged ducts and thrush may occur. The wonderful mother-child bond you expected does not arrive; instead, maternal frustration and depression begin to develop. For your infant, a bloated belly and excessive gas with associated gastrointestinal pain develops, and your baby experiences constant crying, sleepless nights, failure to thrive, and sleep apnea.

CHAPTER 2

The Search for Answers

While still in the hospital, you ask to see a lactation consultant and you speak to your medical doctor. Everyone says, "Oh, you're just a new mother. Everything looks okay. Things will improve in a day or two."

You ask, "Do you think something is wrong? Could my baby be tongue- or lip-tied?" They all look at the baby resting in your arms and say, "There is nothing wrong. There's nothing to indicate the presence of any tongue or lip-tie." Or worse, they say, "Oh, there is only a minor tie, but it will not have any effect on your infant's ability to breastfeed."

You are sent home, confused and concerned. You know something is not quite right, but all of your support systems are dismissing your concerns as those of a new mother.

Some of your friends or relatives even tell you that breastfeeding is not meant to be enjoyable. At your follow-up visits to your primary care physician, you are given no suggestions on why things are going wrong.

You go where everyone goes today to find out why things are not going right: the Internet. You type in "breastfeeding problems," and there it is, in bold print: "Maybe your baby is tongue and lip-tied." Again you seek help from your lactation consultant and primary care physician. Again they say there is a very minor tongue-tie, or they tell you the upper lip doesn't have anything to do with breastfeeding, but you get no help. In fact, they suggest you just use formula.

You are left devastated and weepy, and you begin to suffer post-partum depression.

Comments from parents:

> *Almost six months ago I brought my son in to fix his tongue and lip-tie. I was so concerned about the pain he'd be in that I delayed getting it done. My son was back in my arms and nursing within ten minutes. I figured he was in too much pain*

to really latch on because it didn't hurt! I was thrilled to find out that *breastfeeding doesn't have to hurt and can be really enjoyable.* I was shocked and overjoyed that he instantly had a better latch and no more pain. After three cases of mastitis and a breast abscess from his poor latch, I never thought we'd have such a great breastfeeding relationship. Our only regret is that we did not do it sooner.

* * *

After we discovered our two-month-old was beginning to lose weight, we made the two-hour trip to Dr. Kotlow's office (they got us in the same week). Turns out our daughter was stage 4 100% tongue and lip tied. The surgery took no longer than five minutes, and she was back in our arms. After a few days, she was eating better then ever and has gained almost a pound in less than two weeks! We couldn't be happier and thank Dr. Kotlow and his staff for helping our little girl.

* * *

After two unsuccessful tongue-tie surgeries by an ENT, I was referred to Dr. Kotlow's office by my pediatrician's NP. It was also discovered that he was severely lip-tied as well, which nobody else ever noticed. Dr. Kotlow did an amazing job releasing my son's lip and his tongue. His knowledge in this area is unmatched by any other. He was very fast and efficient. I wish that I was referred to him prior to my son's two failed surgeries. My experience with Dr. Kotlow and his staff is by far the best experience that I have ever had with any medical professional.

* * *

I wanted to sincerely thank Dr. Kotlow for helping correct my daughter's posterior tongue-tie and lip-tie. Thanks to Dr. Kotlow, I have been exclusively nursing for over five months now, after being told by various medical and other professionals that EBF was not a possibility for us. From failure to thrive and nonstop nursing/pumping/supplementing sessions, my eight-month-old daughter is now a chubby, healthy, and superefficient nurser. Working to establish a solid nursing relationship with my daughter was a job that I did not take lightly and worked around the clock to achieve. In the first three months of my daughter's life, I visited countless medical specialists, LCs, cranial-sacral therapists, etc., many of whom implored me to "just give up." While I had heard of Dr. Kotlow from the web and a number of LCs, and my motherly instinct told me early on that we should just get in the car and go see him, I was hesitant to make an appointment because he was so far away, and I thought that I should work with a local ENT first. Well, after a successfully unsuccessful clipping by a local ENT (they only got 50% of the tongue-tie, so all of our nursing issues persisted), and as a last ditch effort to solve our nursing problems; I set out for Albany from NJ. Dr. Kotlow's office was impeccable and state of the art, and he and his staff were kind and extremely considerate and aware of the sensitive state of desperation that mothers like me are in. For a procedure that took less than ten minutes, and a drive that took less than eight hours round trip, the impact that Dr. Kotlow's evaluation/treatment has had on our lives is immeasurable. Thank you, Dr. Kotlow, for giving mothers like me hope, and for giving us a way to support and nourish our children, when most others would just as soon have us give up.

CHAPTER 3

Maternal and Infant Symptoms

As you attempt to bond with your infant through breastfeeding, it becomes a difficult and often painful task. The following symptoms are problems that mothers can and often do develop:

Physical symptoms:

1. Lipstick-shape nipples after the infant latches
2. Flattened, blistered, bruised, cut, or bleeding nipples
3. Moderate to severe pain when your infant attempts to achieve a latch
4. Infected nipples
5. Plugged ducts
6. Mastitis
7. Nipple thrush
8. Engorged or unemptied breasts
9. Premature self-weaning
10. Premature reduction of breast milk supply

Emotional symptoms:

1. Frustration due to lack of answers
2. Exhaustion
3. Depression
4. Lack of infant-mother connection
5. Premature weaning due to pain and frustration
6. Family conflicts and/or unjust accusations from child protective services

Infants who struggle in their attempts to achieve a good latch begin to develop a series of minor and major complications, which are also found in some bottle-fed infants:

1. A short shallow ineffective latch
2. Unsustained latch
3. Sliding off the nipple
4. Prolonged episodes of non-nutritional breastfeeding attempts
5. Unsatisfied nursing episodes
6. Falling asleep before satisfied while attempting to nurse
7. Unable to hold onto a pacifier
8. Poor weight gain, resulting in diagnosis of a failure to thrive infant
9. Chronic crying episodes
10. Can only sleep when held upright or in a car carrier
11. Signs of morning congestion—silent sleeping stomach reflux
12. Infant gastroesophageal reflux
13. Clicking and swallowing air when latched (aerophagia)
14. Leaking milk
15. Hospitalization

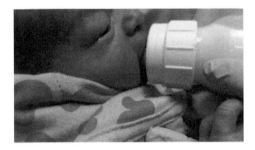

Infants who bottle-feed may exhibit similar symptoms if the latch onto the bottle is also weak and shallow.

CHAPTER 4

Myths v. Facts

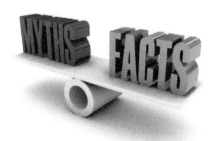

Your baby has been home for a month now, and you are desperately seeking help because of the cascading series of problems, both mental and physical, for you and your newborn. Let's look at the misinformation parents are given by many of the health-care people, friends, and relatives from whom they seek answers to their problems. And let's look at the facts.

MYTH 1: Tongue-ties will correct themselves. The lingual frenum or tongue-tied tongue will stretch or tear without treatment or surgical intervention.

FACT: These ties do not stretch or tear and will remain an interference when attempting to achieve a good secure latch on to the mother's breast.

MYTH 2: The upper lip frenum attachment or maxillary lip-tie has nothing to do with breastfeeding; it is not preventing your infant from achieving a good secure latch.

FACT: When the upper lip fails to elevate or flange upward adequately this may interfere with the infant being able maintain a good secure latch.

MYTH 3: When there is a diagnosis of a lip-tie and/or tongue-tie, you need to wait to revise the ties until your infant is at least one or two years of age.

FACT: Infants who present with tethered oral tissues should and can be treated as early as the day they are born. Waiting does nothing to improve the latch and leads to all the problems discussed earlier in this book.

MYTH 4: Revising tethered oral tissue requires and operating room and general anesthesia.

FACT: The procedure to correct these TOTS can be completed safely, quickly, and easily in a medical or dental office. The procedure—when done correctly, especially using today's laser technology—takes seconds, not minutes to revise.

MYTH 5: The tongue has nothing to do with achieving a good latch and does not interfere with breastfeeding.

FACT: Infants express milk from the mother's breast by creating a vacuum, which occurs when the back of the tongue is free to move up and down untethered. In addition, the tongue must be free to move forward and under the breast nipple to achieve a tight seal and not cause the mother nipple distress and pain.

MYTH 6: There is no such thing as a posterior tongue-tie.

FACT: Tongues that have restricted movements can have attachments at any point on the underside of the tongue from tip all the way back to the base of the tongue. Symptoms determine whether the tongue would benefit from a revision rather than the position of the frenum attachment. As I will discuss later, tongue-ties can be described by appearance as well as lack of function. Determining whether to release the tie involves consideration of many factors, not just breastfeeding.

MYTH 7: Tongue-ties do not cause maternal discomfort.

FACT: A short or restricted tongue can prevent an infant from achieving a tight seal and effective latch. This can result in pain and biting of the nipple, which does indeed create a painful latch.

MYTH 8: Tongue-ties do not exist.

FACT: Tongue-ties can vary in the location of the frenum attachment. They only require revisions when they interfere with normal function or have the potential to create problems in the future such as speech impediments, dental decay, or malocclusions.

MYTH 9: Release or revision the lingual attachment is dangerous due to bleeding or cutting nerves or glands.

FACT: The release or revision of the lingual frenum is a very safe, simple, and quick surgical procedure easily completed in an out-patient setting. Bleeding or damage to other oral structures, when performed by a properly trained surgeon, is not a concern.

MYTH 10: Release of the lingual frenum may cause an infant to choke or swallow his or her tongue. If you cut the tissue the baby can suffocate and die.

FACT: This is not a concern. In fact, it is not even a potential problem since it is not possible. There is no historical information or peer-reviewed scientific articles to substantiate or support this statement.

MYTH 11: Children will fall and fix a maxillary lip-tie, and therefore it does not require any surgical intervention.

FACT: Although this is a possible occurrence, it is not a medical treatment and should not be suggested as a treatment modality. In addition, it is not a potential occurrence for an infant, and it would *in no way* assist in achieving a good latch when breastfeeding. In infants who breastfeed after the eruption of the upper front teeth, a severe lip-tie can trap mother's milk in the folds of the upper lip and potentially lead to facial decay on these teeth. In older children, revising the upper lip benefits the child by preventing tooth decay and formation of a gap between the two front teeth.

MYTH 12: When releasing or revising TOTs, infants will pull out any stitches required.

FACT: Release and revision of these tissues do not require stitches or any type of tacking down.

MYTH13: The mouth is so dirty. Cutting the attachments may lead to an infection.

FACT: The chance of any type of oral infection when revising or releasing these tissues is almost non-existent. In completing over ten thousand revisions, the author has never seen any type of infection due to soft tissue surgical procedures.

MYTH 14: Surgical correction of these tissues using a laser is dangerous; it can burn or cause an explosion.

FACT: Lasers have been available for oral surgery since the late nineties and are completely safe for any age or patient. They do not burn or cause explosions and are safe, quick, and effective. They often do not require any type of numbing for the surgery and heal uneventfully.

MYTH 15: Post-surgical exercises are too difficult and stressful for parents.

FACT: Partially true for some parents. When done correctly these post-surgical wound management procedures are quick and relatively easy to accomplish. Parents need to understand that they are breastfeeding for all the scientifically proven benefits. Not unlike a broken arm when the cast comes off, post-injury physical therapy is needed to relearn proper function and mobility, and the same is true for post-revision soft tissue surgical care.

MYTH 16: The only reason anyone uses a laser is to pay for it. Lasers are dangerous to use on infants.

FACT: This is an unfortunate comment made by non-laser dentists who lack any scientific understanding of lasers and how they are used in dentistry and medicine. In fact, lasers are the state of the art in both hard- and soft-tissue dental surgery today. The cost of any laser is not a factor in providing our patients the best dental care available today.

MYTH17: In order to release a tongue-tie a Z-Plasty is required.

FACT: A Z-Plasty or major surgical procedure is rarely required in revising an infant's tongue-tie.

MYTH 18: You should just wait and everything will be okay, or you can just use a bottle and formula.

FACT: If you want to breastfeed your infant, then waiting months for resolution of the problems is not a recognized prudent medical treatment. Infants using a bottle with tethered oral tissues may still have difficulties similar to those experienced by infants who breastfeed. *Formula does not provide the infant the same health or structural benefits as breastfeeding.*

MYTH 19: An infant's latch has nothing to do with infant acid reflux.

FACT: Infants rarely have true gastroesophageal reflux disease (GERD) and are often treated with adult acid reflux drugs to alleviate the problem with little or no success or benefit. Infant reflux is often misdiagnosed and treated inappropriately when in fact it is due to the infant not achieving a good latch and swallowing air. This is known as aerophagia.

MYTH 20: Infant sleep apnea has nothing to do with tongue-ties.

FACT: Infant sleep apnea results in reduced oxygen for the brain and the rapidly developing nervous system during the first year of life. This is being studied as a cause of attention-deficit/hyperactivity disorder, among other things. A tongue that is significantly tethered cannot move forward, so when the infant is placed on his or her back, it may cause the tongue to fall backward and block the infant's airway, thus leading to sleep apnea.

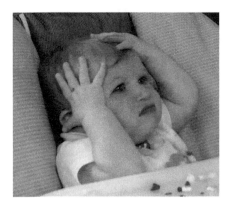

These comments/myths are based on unsupported as well as undocumented information and make it confusing and often difficult for mothers to get appropriate care for their infant. The failure to breastfeed is often placed on the mother, although it is most likely due to the infant's lip and tongue attachments.

CHAPTER 5

Why Breastfeeding is Beneficial

"Breastfeeding and human milk are the normative standards for infant feeding and nutrition. Given the documented short- and long-term medical and neurodevelopmental advantages of breastfeeding, infant nutrition should be considered a public health issue and not only a lifestyle choice."

PEDIATRICS Vol. 129 No. 3 March 1, 2012 pp. e827 -e841 (doi: 10.1542/peds.2011-3552)

Making the decision to breastfeed your infant is a personal and important choice you make when your infant is born. Since it is a personal choice, some mothers who choose not to breastfeed or are unable to breastfeed for medical or physical complications should not be criticized.

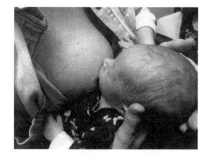

The American Academy of Pediatrics in their March 2013 policy on breastfeeding states, "Breastfeeding should not be considered as a lifestyle choice, but rather as a basic health issue."

On the same question, Jane Morgan, MD, states, "Unquestionably, breast milk is far superior to any formula designed for babies, and even more critical for the health of the premature baby. The challenge lies in making breastfeeding, or providing a mother's own milk for her baby, a comfortable, enjoyable, and manageable part of the new mother's life."

In 2012 the surgeon general of the United States stated, "For nearly all infants, breastfeeding is the best source of infant nutrition and immunologic protection, and it provides remarkable health benefits to mothers as well. Babies who are breastfed are less likely to become overweight and obese."

The Secretary of the US Department of Health and Human Services concluded that, "As one of the most universal and natural facets of motherhood, the ability to breastfeed is a great gift. Breastfeeding helps mothers and babies bond, and it is vitally important to mothers' and infants' health. *For much of the last century, America's mothers were given poor advice and were discouraged from breastfeeding, to the point that breastfeeding became an unusual choice in this country.*

However, in recent decades, as mothers, their families, and health professionals have realized the importance of breastfeeding, the desire of mothers to breastfeed has soared. More and more mothers are breastfeeding every year. In fact, over three-quarters of all newborns in America now begin their lives breastfeeding, and breastfeeding has regained its rightful place in our nation as the norm—the way most mothers feed their newborns.

In addition to all the known health benefits that breastfeeding produces, we also know that breastfed infants benefit in the development of the oral, facial, muscular, and skeletal development when breastfeeding rather than bottle-feeding

American Academy of Pediatrics New Mother's Guide to Breastfeeding (2011) suggests the following benefits to breastfeeding your infant and mothers

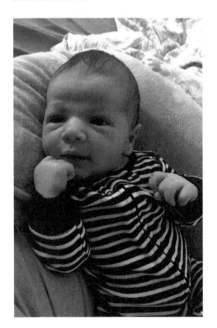

Infant benefits

1. Benefits an infant's overall immune system
2. Allergy prevention
3. Breast milk has no added preservatives always fresh: a great homemade meal
4. Development of emotional attachment between parents and infant
5. Protect against gastroenteritis, constipation, and other stomach illnesses
6. Reduced risks of sleep apnea, SIDS, behavior problems in toddlers

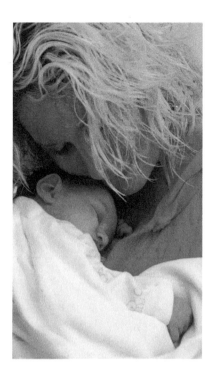

Maternal benefits

1. Assists in maternal fulfillment
2. Reduces risks for breast cancer
3. Reduces risks for uterine and ovarian cancers
4. Reduces risks for type 2 diabetes, rheumatoid arthritis and cardiovascular disease
5. Lessens osteoporosis
6. Promotes emotional health—body and mind—and can prevent post-partum depression
7. Promotes post-partum weight loss

Economic and environmental benefits

1. Fewer sick days off for mothers
2. Less energy and waste for manufacturing formula
3. Cost savings—if all mothers breastfed exclusively for the first six months—$13 billion a year

CHAPTER 6

When, Where and to Whom Do You Go to Make the Diagnosis?

There are many unfortunate barriers for mothers getting good sound advice and a diagnosis of tongue-ties and lip-ties as the cause of their maternal and infant breastfeeding difficulties.

The first problem, and one of the most difficult, is changing old medical concepts—believing that doing no treatment is better than doing any surgical treatment. Often the medical Hippocratic Oath of "doing no harm" is misrepresented as just watching and waiting. The concept of medically necessary care is the first hurdle we need to jump over.

As defined by the American Academy of Pediatric Dentistry in their guidelines, **medically necessary care** (MNC) is the reasonable and **appropriate** diagnostic, **preventive** treatment services and follow-up care as determined by qualified, appropriate health-care providers in treating **any condition**, including a disease, an injury, or a congenital or developmental malformation. In addition, it states that medically necessary care includes all supportive health-care services that, in the judgment of the attending dentist, are necessary for the provision of optimal quality **therapeutic and preventive oral care.**

Thus we can reasonably say that revising the lip- and tongue-ties in infants with symptoms of breastfeeding difficulties meets the requirement of a congenital or developmental malformation requiring a therapeutic and preventive intervention for optimal oral care.

The second significant barrier to treatment is the medical community's reluctance to understand the idea of evidence-based knowledge and how it can be assimilated into the concept of *scientific plausibility*.

Scientific plausibility can—and often should—be substituted for the concept of evidence-based knowledge when we look at the accumulated experience, education, and clinical skills of many practitioners who have been revising infants' TOTs for years with great success.

- When an infant is in pain due to reflux or presents failure to thrive, is this better treated by doing nothing or by surgical intervention?
- And when mothers who cannot bond with their infants due to being unable to breastfeed and in consequence suffer from post-partum depression, when they resort to pumping to maintain adequate breast supply to provide their infants with breast milk, is this better treated by doing nothing or by surgical intervention?

The answer to both questions is obvious: surgical intervention and revising or releasing these tissues is better for the infant and the mother than doing nothing.

Once we accept the idea of revision as an alternative to doing nothing, the next step is to find out when, where, and to whom you go for the correct diagnosis and referral for care.

When women have difficulties attempting breastfeeding, they are often confronted with two divergent paths. Well-meaning lactation consultants urge them to try harder, and some doctors might advise them to simply stop trying to breastfeed and use the bottle. Then they hand the mothers free samples of formula.

When you think tethered oral tissues are the cause for infant and maternal problems, you as a parent have a dilemma that confronts you. Lactation and breastfeeding are the only human functions that do not routinely have medical training, medical procedures or residency programs where physicians or dentists can learn and understand differential diagnostic ways to help you.

Modern medicine has not been able to decide where breastfeeding problems should be addressed. Since breasts are partially where the problems are observed, is it the OB/GYN physician who should be treating the problem? Or since it is the infant who presents with the problems and indeed is the real source of the problem, does the pediatrician or family practice physician assume the responsibility? All too often neither is equipped to do so. The result is that mothers continue to suffer, and nothing really changes.

In the hospital, right after the infant is delivered, many mothers see a lactation consultant. In most hospitals, this person is generally an IBCLC or international board certified lactation consultant, although others may be just partially trained lactation consultants. If you have delivered at home, your midwife may be your source of support.

Often because of the pressure from medical doctors, who are not sympathetic to the concept of tongue- and lip-ties, if these hospital-based consultants examine your infant the hospital, the "GAG or be fired" rule prevents them from even suggesting to you that the oral tissues may be the source of your symptoms. They cannot urge you to seek an evaluation and possible release or revision of the tongue- and upper lip-ties. In essence, the hospital physicians feel that only a trained physician or dentist can make the diagnosis.

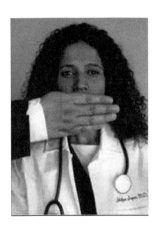

The hospital silent "gag or be fired" rule

It is a poorly kept secret worldwide that IBCLCs, nurses, and other non-medical personnel who are hospital employees and who might suggest to a mother that her infant is possibly tongue-tied may result in the person losing his or her job.

The breastfeeding team

In an ideal world, we would have a "breastfeeding team." The breastfeeding team would consist of the delivery room nurse or midwife for home births, followed by the pediatrician or family practice physician, the IBCLC, often a body worker such as an infant chiropractor or cranial-sacral therapist and the pediatric or family practice dentist.

The first step in making a correct diagnosis

Where and when can the initial evaluation be made? The initial evaluation of whether your infant might have any difficulties achieving a good latch should begin within the first few hours of life. When your infant is born, he or she is usually placed on your belly to begin the mother-infant bonding. Infants instinctively know where to go. They migrate right to your breast, looking for nourishment.

Once this bonding begins, a simple finger sweep across the floor of the mouth can help indicate if breastfeeding is going to be problematical or be a wonderful beginning. This can be performed by a trained nurse in the delivery room, in the nursery, or at the mother's bedside. But it's ideal to wait for the initial mother-infant bond to have some time to occur.

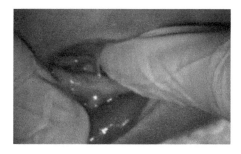

Place your index finger into the area where the lower molars will eventually erupt and pass it across the floor of the mouth. The initial finger sweep is checking for any degree of soft tissue interference or obstruction, which can indicate a potential problem when the mother begins to breastfeed.

Evaluating the tongue sweep

After evaluating under the tongue for any type of obstruction, an examiner's finger should be placed gently into the infant's mouth so the infant's suck can be evaluated.

A shallow latch can result in gum pad pressure or discomfort on the examiner's fingernail and may cause the infant to gag because of the tongue's inability to extend forward and pass under the fingertip. This is caused when a restrictive tongue-tie reduces the ability of the tongue to protrude forward and not block the infant's airway. Tongue thrusting is another problem to look for and occurs when an infant pushes his/her tongue outward, pushing the breast away and interfering with latching on.

A smooth uninterrupted pass under the tongue.	Most likely the infant will not have difficulties achieving a successful latch.
A slight interrupted pass or significant interference under the tongue.	The mother should be made aware of the types of symptoms to be looking for when the infant attempts to latch.
A small, medium, or large piece of membranous mucosal tissue interfering with the finger sweep.	Almost always will interfere with the infant's ability to achieve an adequate latch. Mothers need to be advised of the symptoms to look for.
A thin or thick piece of membranous tissue attaching close to the tip of the tongue, obstructing the ability to allow a finger sweep. An appearance of a heart-shaped tongue.	These should alert the assessing person that the attachment should be revised immediately, before symptoms develop.

An adequate latch—or a latch achieved after a successful revision—will allow for the tongue to slide under the fingernail, eliminating or preventing any gagging, as well as producing a gentle massaging action on the area of the finger above the fingernail between the first and second knuckle. The gagging is a result of the tongue's inability to extend forward and pass under the fingertip, caused when a restrictive tongue-tie reduces the ability of the tongue to protrude forward and not block the infant's airway. Tongue thrusting is another problem to look for and occurs when an infant pushes his/her tongue outward, pushing the breast away and interfering with latching on.

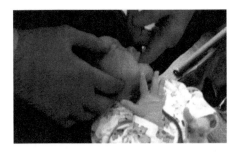 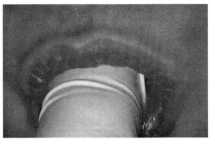

Place your index finger into the infant's mouth and allow the infant to suck on the finger. A shallow latch will place pressure on the fingernail and cause discomfort. It may also cause the infant to gag, due to forcing the tongue backward into the infant's airway.

IBCLC—international board-certified lactation consultant

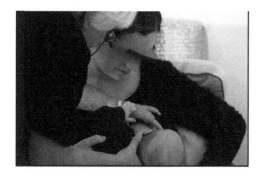

The next person to see a mother and infant will most likely be the IBCLC or lactation consultant. The consultant should check the infant for any interferences, assist a mother on the most effective position for the infant to achieve a good latch, and check the oral structures for any signs of restrictive attachments.

The consultant should ideally be able to suggest to a mother that if problems are occurring or if they begin to occur, she should see someone for a revision. In an ideal situation the consultant will suggest to also possibly see a bodyworker, such as a chiropractor or cranial-sacral therapist, to help relax the infant's head and neck structures. This also aids in the correct diagnosis and can help if these are contributing factors to the breastfeeding problems. However, I do not recommend a long drawn-out course of therapy prior to revisions.

The wait-and-see recommendation

Insurance may not cover additional bodywork, and since it is often expensive, parents may skip this important step. Breastfeeding will not be successful without the oral tissues being revised or released. Waiting and doing nothing is not a practical solution, especially if you are the one suffering from pain and discomfort, and your infant is not well-nourished.

Once a diagnosis of restricted oral tissues is made, your infant should be seen as quickly as possible to avoid further damage to your breast and nipples and for your infant's nutrition.

Where to go for treatment

Where can you go for the surgical release or revision of the lip- and tongue-tie? In some instances, your options are quite limited, and in other instances, you may have a list of potential options.

The quick snip

The first option, which I recommend you avoid if at all possible, is the so-called "quick snip." This is when any physician takes a pair of scissors and releases a few millimeters of tissue under the tongue. In almost all instances, this is an incomplete, insufficient, and inadequate release of the tissue. In addition, this person will rarely examine, evaluate, or even recognize the need to revise or release the upper lip-tie. Resolution of the symptoms is delayed and you still need to see someone for further treatment.

The ENT and the operating room

The next option is often a referral from the primary care physician to an ear, nose, and throat specialist (ENT) physician. Usually the same procedure occurs—a quick snip with a pair of scissors—and an assurance to you that the upper lip has no effect on achieving a good latch. If the ENT agrees that these tissues need to be released or revised, he or she often suggests waiting until the infant is older and/or then doing the procedure in an operating room under a general anesthetic.

This option doesn't address the immediate problems and will often lead to premature weaning to the bottle, but with the infant's symptoms remaining. Placing an infant under general anesthesia at this age is neither recommended nor necessary when other options are far safer and less invasive.

The laser option

I recommend seeking someone trained and educated in the use of surgical soft-tissue dental lasers. Laser revisions are quick, safe, and easily completed in a few minutes in a dental office or the office of a physician who is trained in laser surgery. If a laser surgeon is not available, I recommend seeking out a well-trained person who understands lip- and tongue-ties and can be effective in properly revising or releasing them *if scissors are only option.*

Electrosurgical releases are also an option, but this is a burn and should only be an option if a laser is not available. If a surgeon is routinely revising or releasing tethered oral tissues, there is no excuse for not investing in and using a laser for the benefit of his or her patients. A more in-depth discussion of the surgery and diagnosis will follow in this book.

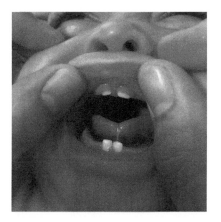

In almost all infants suffering from tethered oral tissues that interfere with a secure latch, the upper lip-tie's failure to elevate during the infant's attempts to latch and the restricted tongue work together to prevent successful breastfeeding. Revising one without the other will usually result in continued breastfeeding difficulties.

CHAPTER 7
Tongue-Ties (Ankyloglossia)

Breastfeeding requires the synchronized coordination of the jaws, tongue and lips and of course mother's breast.

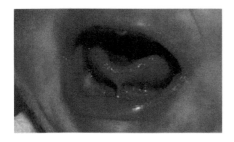

Ankyloglossia or Tongue-tied

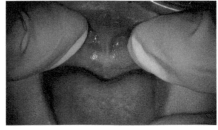

The maxillary lip tie

The tongue-tie, or ankyloglossia

The tissue under the tongue, which attaches the tongue to the floor of the mouth, is known as the lingual frenum. The International Affiliation of Tongue-Tie Professionals (IATP) defines a tongue-tie as *the embryologic remnant of the tissue in the midline of the undersurface of the tongue and the floor of the mouth.*

Expanding that definition further, I add that a tongue-tie is an (*abnormal*) attachment of the membrane that fastens the tongue to the floor of the mouth, which may interfere with the normal mobility and function of the tongue.

Our tongue is an amazing muscle. It is the only muscle in our body that is attached at one end and at the other end to eight other muscles. The unattached end is usually free to move in almost any direction untethered. If the tongue is prevented from untethered movement, however, it can have a cascading effect on almost every organ system in our body and create oral dysfunction syndrome.

When this muscle is prevented in utero from elevating and molding the hard palate, it may prevent the maxillary hard palate from expanding upward and laterally, giving way to the formation of a high-arch palate.

This high-arched palate often results in preventing the nipple from getting far enough into the oral cavity to achieve a good latch; it also contributes to the development of a malocclusion in the future (improper bite or upper and lower jaw development), and since the top of the hard palate represents the floor of the maxillary sinus, a tethered tongue can also affect our infant's maxillary sinus development. Thus, a restricted or tethered tongue has the potential to affect skeletal growth and development.

As I have mentioned, if the tongue is restricted from moving forward and remains tethered to the floor of the mouth, it can lead to the blocking of an infant's airway, which may cause sleep apnea. It may affect respiration, cause insufficient oxygenation, and hamper ideal neurologic development, thus affecting the neuromuscular, respiratory, cardiac and nervous systems. When it interferes with achieving a good latch on a mother's breast, it can affect the nutrition of the infant, promote air-induced reflux and harm the digestive system.

It also eventually can affect dental development, be a source of TMJ problems and pain (temporomandibular jaw dysfunction) and head-aches, and contribute to dental decay as the infant develops.

Diagnosing a tongue-tie—the initial examination

Identifying lip and tongue problems requires placing the infant into the correct examination position. In order to adequately evaluate the infant's oral structures, the infant's head should be positioned in the examiner's lap so that it faces the same direction as the examiner.

Trying to evaluate an infant while it is moving and sitting on the mother's lap hinders the ability to make a proper diagnosis.

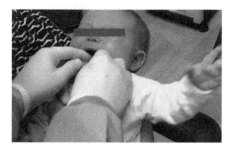

Many infant lip and tongue-ties are missed or misdiagnosed due to improperly examining the infant. This allows the infant to become uncontrollable during the examination while in a mother's arms. It is difficult to see the inside of the oral cavity and properly evaluate all of the structures.

In the delivery room, the infant can be examined in the infant warmer and thereafter using the knee-to-knee position. In the knee-to-knee position, a mother can control the feet and hands while the infant is resting, stabilized, in her lap. This allows an excellent visualization of the entire oral cavity and its structures, and it allows the mother to see exactly what you are seeing.

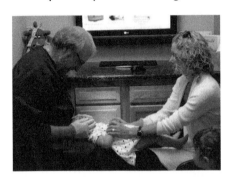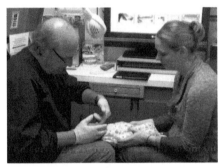

No matter what age, newborns to age three, this is the best position to examine the child.

The next two criteria, which are beneficial in making the right diagnoses, are based on evaluating the clinical location of the insertion point of the lingual attachment to the underside of the infant's tongue and the tongue's ability to move—up and down, forward and backward easily, or with difficulty due to restriction.

The following classifications use the insertion points or attachment locations of the tongue and lip and should be part of the IBCLC oral examination.

Kotlow classifications of the tongue-tie in infants

The author created a simple and quick tongue classification that designates the area in front of the salivary duct as a Class IV tongue-tie when located closest to the tip, or a Class III tongue-tie if closer to the anterior part of the salivary duct.

When the attachment is located distal, or behind, the duct, the area just behind the duct is a Class II tie, and the area closest to the base of the tongue is a Class I tie. Class I ties can also be identified as submucosal ties if they are buried into the base of the tongue.

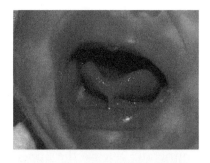

Class IV tongue-tie located at the tip of the tongue and extending halfway between the salivary duct and tip of the tongue. It is the most limiting type of attachment and is often "snipped" by a pair of scissors leaving behind the remaining tie as a posterior tie. A complete revision should extend to the base of the tongue.

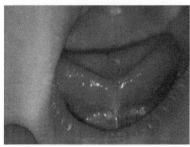

Class III tongue-tie is located in front of the salivary duct halfway to the tip of the tongue. This type of attachment is as significant as a class IV tie and requires release as far back as the base of the tongue.

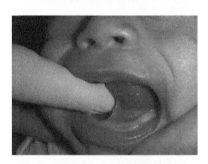

Class II tongue-tie is located between the back of the salivary duct halfway to the base of the tongue.

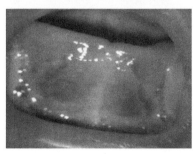

Class I tongue-tie is located from the base of the tongue halfway to the salivary duct.

Anterior and posterior tongue-ties

A confusing set of terms used by some to describe a tongue-tie suggests using the term **anterior tongue-tie** or a **posterior tongue-tie.**

What is not understood by most people who use this designation is that every anterior tongue-tie has, as part of its attachment, a posterior component. This leads to many incomplete or partial revisions or release of the lingual frenum.

This seems especially true when the surgeon uses scissors for the release or revision, just snipping the portion anteriorly and not completing the release, leaving the posterior portion of the attachment intact. This accompanies a failure to examine and release the upper lip-tie. The position of the tie is described as located either anterior or posterior to the submandibular salivary duct, which is located in the floor of the mouth.

Any attachment forward of the salivary duct would therefore be considered an anterior tie and attachment behind the salivary duct is identified as a posterior tie. In either way to facilitate elimination of the breastfeeding difficulties the lingual frenum attachment needs to be released completely to the base of the tongue.

The submucosal or true posterior tongue-tie

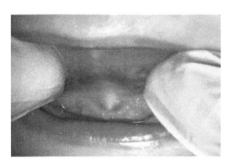
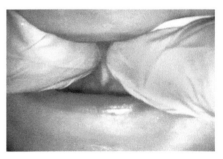
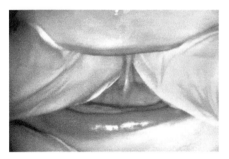

The submucosal or posterior class I tongue-tie can become more pronounced when the examination is completed in the examiner's lap and the index fingers are placed at the insertion point and pressed downward. This will usually elevate the tie and make it more visible.

Successful identification of a submucosal or posterior attachment is only possible when viewing the infant in the knee-to-knee position and pushing down on the frenum to allow the attachment to pop out.

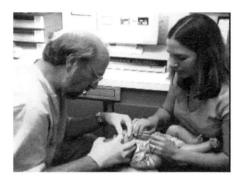

Thrush or Just Dried Milk?

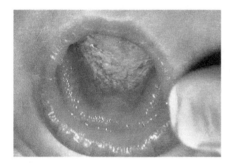 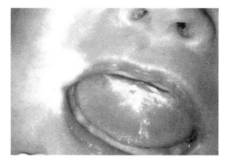

Incorrect diagnosis of infant oral thrush is often an inaccurate medical diagnosis when in fact it is caused by milk being trapped on the upper surface of the infant's tongue. This will usually come right off when using a toothbrush on the tongue's surface.

CHAPTER 8

The Maxillary Lip-Tie

The maxillary lip-tie

Definition: A remnant of the tissue in the midline of the upper lip and the gum that holds the lip attached to the gum (gingiva), which may interfere with the normal mobility and function of the upper lip, contributing to poor latch by the infant onto the breast.

In addition, in some cases, when mothers elect to breastfeed at will during the night without cleaning off the teeth after nursing, the lip-tie may contribute to decay formation on the front surfaces of the upper central and lateral incisor teeth.

If an infant is born with any oral soft-tissue abnormalities or variations, breastfeeding may become difficult. One variation that is often overlooked occurs when the upper lip is too tightly attached to the maxillary gingival tissue.

This band of tissue is known as the superior labial frenum, the median labial frenum, or the maxillary labial frenum. This is a portion of mucous membrane containing loose connective tissue. It may insert into the maxillary arch's free gingival tissue or the attached gingival tissue. In more severe instances, the tissue may be connected into the area of the incisive papilla.

In addition to the ability of the tongue to function in achieving a successful latch, the maxillary lip should be free to enable the infant's lip to extend upward to maximize the infant's attachment onto the areola, rather than onto just the nipple.

When the upper lip's inner (soft-tissue) mucosa is attached to the alveolar ridge of the maxillary arch (upper jaw) and the lip is unable to fully flange upward, it is a factor in creating a shallow latch.

The following criteria are used to classify and evaluate the upper lip attachment. The upper lip can be classified by assessing the inner lip's mucosal attachment. When the lip attachment inserts into the zone where the two upper front teeth will emerge and extends beyond the maxillary alveolar ridge into the palatal area, the lip-tie is classified as a class IV lip-tie. When it inserts into the zone just forward of the palatal area between the area of the future two front teeth it is a class III lip-tie. The insertion zone into the area of the free and attached gingiva is identified as a class II lip-tie, and if the attachment is above this area, it is identified as class I.

Kotlow Classification of the Lip-Tie in Infants

Location of the lip-tie is based on the zone of attachment of the inner lip's mucosa.

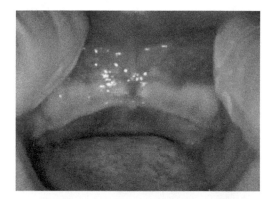

Class I lip-tie. This is the least common location and is not commonly seen in infants.

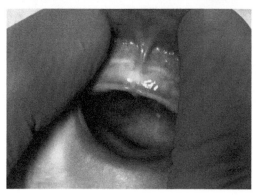

Class II lip-tie, inserting at the zone of the free and attached gingival tissue. A very commonly found attachment which can easily be enough of a tie to prevent the full extension of the upper lip and allow a tight attachment of the infant on the mother's breast.

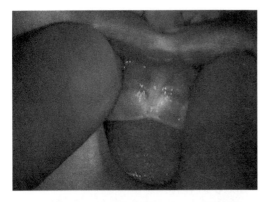

Class III lip-tie inserting at the zone between the areas of the future central incisors. This can be a significant attachment in limiting the upper lips ability to successfully flange upward.

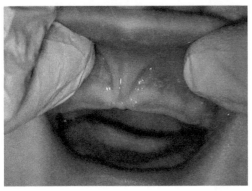

Class IV lip-tie, inserting at the zone extending into the anterior palatal area. This attachment is not only going to interfere with a mother's ability to successfully latch but also may contribute to a large gap between the upper front teeth, dental decay, and pain.

The nursing blister or lip callous

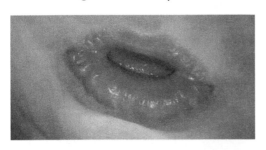

The presence of lip calluses or lip blisters are an additional sign that the upper lip is not elevating well and causing the tissue to be irritated, thus producing blister lip lesions.

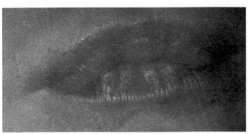

CHAPTER 9

Dental Decay and At-Will Nighttime Breastfeeding

Dental decay on the upper front teeth

In 1977, it was first reported that some infants who were exclusively nursing presented with a pattern of anterior decay different from decay observed in children who were allowed to sleep or rest with a baby bottle containing liquids other than water.

Differential diagnostic discussions with nursing mothers indicated that these infants were receiving nutrition entirely from breast milk, and that in most instances were sleeping with the mother and engaging in at-will nursing. Two to three times during the night the infant nursed, a feeding pattern that continued after the eruption of the upper and lower central and lateral incisors, and in some cases beyond the age of two or three after upper cuspids and molars had erupted

The pattern of decay seen in baby-bottle caries usually presents as lingual caries on the upper central and lateral incisors, followed by decay of the upper first molars.

Infants who breastfeed and are born with an abnormal maxillary frenum attachment often present with a different pattern of dental caries—facial caries on the upper incisors—that often appears as either facial decay or incisal notching.

Breastfeeding alone doesn't cause dental decay. However, when the upper lip-tie is present, and this tie is left tethered, then during at-will nighttime nursing once the upper front teeth erupt, dental decay may be produced when the upper lip-tie interferes with removal of residual milk during the night.

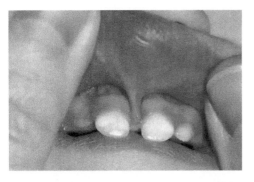

Initial beginning stages of tooth enamel decalcification or decay.

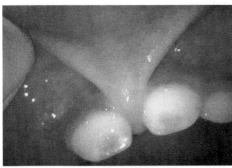

Enamel decay progression.

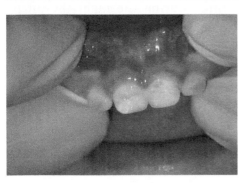

Moderate decay on the front or facial surfaces of the upper front teeth.

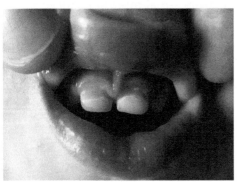

Extensive decay formation on the front or facial surfaces of the upper front teeth.

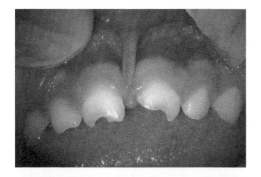

Incisal edges of upper front teeth developing notching decay patterns.

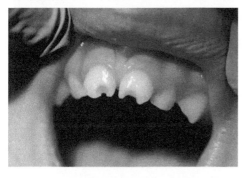

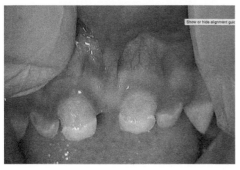

Severe decay development on the upper front teeth.

Treating these problems includes release of the maxillary lip-tie, restoring the teeth, and the use of a topical fluoride gel to assist in rematerializing pre-decay areas.

CHAPTER 10

The Other Ties—Buccal and Mandibular Ties

The other tethered tissues that may contribute to poor latching and efficient breastfeeding, include tight maxillary or upper arch buccal attachments, as well as tight lingual and buccal mandibular alveolar ridge attachments.

During the infant's initial oral examination, running your index finger between the upper cheek between the area in the maxillary arch where the future first and second primary molars will eventually erupt may find small strands of tight tissue called the buccal frenum which may prevent the cheeks from moving in and out and also interfere with the infant's ability to achieve a good latch.

A tight mandibular buccal and/or lingual alveolar ridge attachment may interfere with the lower lip from flanging downward and thus also interfere with a tight latch.

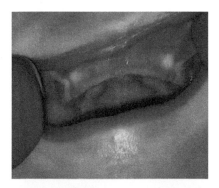

During the knee-to-knee oral examination the examiner should pull the cheeks outward and feel for any tight frenum like attachment of the cheek to the maxillary or mandibular gingival tissue. This is usually in the first primary molar-cuspid region. These are identified as "BUCCAL" frenum attachments.

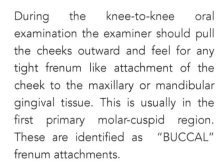

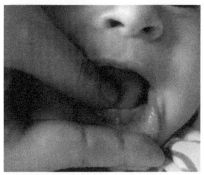

When an infant attaches to the breast the lower lip also will flange downward allowing the baby to successfully attach. When it is observed not allowing a good attachment, it may also require a release.

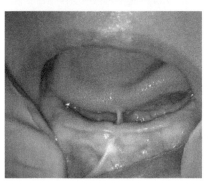

Occasionally the lingual attachment has two separate areas of attachment. The normal lingual tie and a further anterior tie to the mandibular alveolar gingiva tissue. They may need release, but should not be released first as often it disappears when a normal release is completed. Care should be taken with either of the above releases since the areas are very vascular and unless a laser is used the area may bleed.

CHAPTER 11

Abnormalities of the Breasts or Nipples

In addition to the infant oral tissue attachment problems, we should evaluate and diagnose the clinical appearance of the mother's breasts or nipples, which can also be a significant factor in preventing the infant's latch. These may be attributed to the mother's breast anatomy, prior surgeries, and nipple piercing.

Breast anatomy

The anatomy of the breast becomes a problem when the infant has a relatively small mouth and the mother has excessively large nipples or breasts, inverted or short nipples, breast reduction surgery, or a low milk supply.

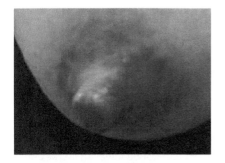

Some mothers present with very large breasts and/or large nipples. These anatomic situations may represent an additional roadblock for infants with very small mouths and may take a while for the infant to grow and enable a good latch. Often seeing an IBCLC can provide alternative infant positioning to overcome these problems.

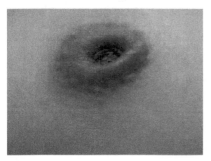

An additional challenge for both the mother and the infant occurs when mother's nipples are either inverted or very small. Nipple shields or other measures suggested by the IBCLC will usually enable a mother to overcome these problems.

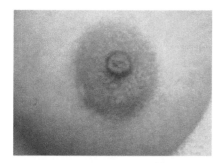

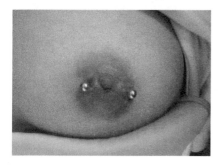

Piercing of the nipple may produce scarring and prevent proper milk release during latch.

Nipple trauma

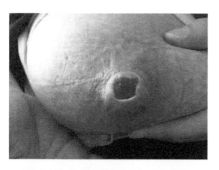

Damaged nipples : In instances where breastfeeding has been attempted and the tethered tongue, lip. or other issues have not been revised, this may lead to significant pain and damage to a mother's nipple. This unfortunately may also lead to premature weaning due to severe toe-curling maternal pain.

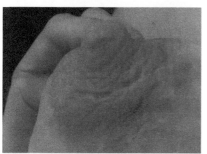

When an infant's latch is borderline, once the infant's upper front teeth begin to erupt, the latch may become painful when the teeth start biting the mother's breast.

PART 2

The following chapters are more technical. They are beneficial for some interested parents who are looking for additional information and for health-care professionals treating infants with TOTs.

CHAPTER 12

Choosing the Best Surgical Treatment

Scissors, Electrosurgery, or Lasers

Historical method for the release of a tongue-tie

The concept of treating and diagnosing tongue-ties is not something new, nor is it a fad in today's world. In the beginning of life as we know it, those infants who could not achieve a good latch would have most likely died if they were not able to get proper nourishment. It was survival of the fittest. In the Bible, Mark 7:32–37 states that he enabled a man to speak by grasping his tongue and once he released the binding and loosened his tongue he could speak.

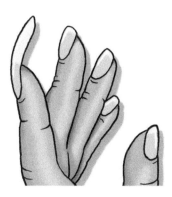

Centuries ago, midwives used their sharpened fingernails to release the tethered tongue. As we learned about infection and asepsis, this method of surgery was pushed aside.

Deciding on whom, where and when to revise or release your infant's tethered oral tissues

Once your infant has been examined and diagnosed, you need to make an informed decision on how, whom and where you want the tongue and lip revised.

Seek out an experienced surgeon who has treated many infants with breastfeeding issues and has a clear understanding of how the tethered oral tissues work to provide a good seal on a mother's breast and thus allow for a secure trouble free latch.

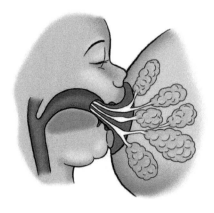

In order to achieve a good effective latch, the tongue must move up and down in the posterior portion. A tethered tongue cannot do this, and the result is ineffective and non-nutritional nursing.

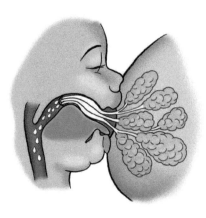

The mechanism that allows the infant to express milk from the breast is a vacuum. This vacuum is produced by the action of the posterior portion of the tongue moving up and the tongue's interaction with the soft palate. The infant will take around 8–12 sucks, stop for 2–3 seconds to swallow, and then repeat the process.

Scissors revisions or partial incomplete releases

Although there are many competent surgeons using scissors to release or revise the lip and tongue, today's state-of-the-art treatment is using a dental laser to ablate soft tissue. Unless there is no option to invest in a laser, anyone who is routinely revising these infants, toddlers, teens, and adults should be fully invested in obtaining and using lasers.

Incomplete scissor releases or revisions of the tethered tongue.

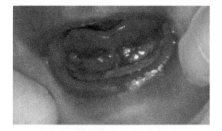

Incomplete revision created a posterior attachment a day after release with scissors. Failure to extend the revision to the base of the tongue results in two problems. One, incomplete release of the attachment, and two, the need for additional surgery to fully release the attachment.

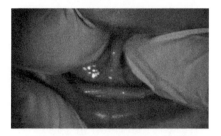

The incomplete or short "snip" of the anterior portion of the lingual frenum attachment serves little purpose except to create a posterior tie. This release was completed a day earlier by a surgeon using a pair of scissors without any improvement in the breastfeeding problems.

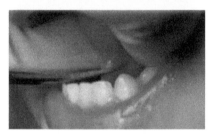

This is an example of the surgeon only partially releasing the lingual attachment using a pair of scissors. Note the "snip" does not fully allow the tongue to achieve complete mobility.

CHAPTER 13

Lasers and Oral Surgery

A brief history of lasers in oral surgery

In 1962 a dermatologist named Leon Goldman came up with a way to remove unwanted tattoos. Utilizing new breakthroughs in laser technology, Dr. Goldman applied a laser to the tattooed area, and presto, the tattoo disappeared. Dr. Goldman's experiment was the first use of lasers in medical history. Since Dr. Goldman first used a laser to remove a tattoo, lasers have become an integral part of modern medicine. The first laser specifically designed for dentistry was marketed in 1989.

A variety of laser wavelengths are available for dentistry. In the United States, the US Food and Drug Administration regulates laser manufacturers. All currently available hot dental lasers have indications for use for incising, excising, and coagulating oral soft-tissue surgery and erbium and CO_2 @9300 for both hard- and soft-tissue treatments.

Since the late nineties, there has been a plethora of research in dental laser applications. The use of the dental lasers has been proved to be an effective tool to increase efficiency, specificity, ease, cost, and comfort of the dental treatment. Dental lasers have been available for oral surgery since 1994; they are extremely safe, fast, and effective.

General anesthesia or in the office

Parents and physicians of newborn infants should be reluctant to place any infant into an operating room and have a general anesthetic for an elective procedure. Unfortunately sometimes this is often the only option available to parents when an infant requires the revision of tethered oral tissues.

Correcting these problems in the dental surgery/office or medical office with a laser has many advantages over those methods. Lasers are bactericidal, usually bloodless, do not require placement of sutures, anesthetic-free, fast, and a safe alternative for infants.

The American Academy of Pediatric Dentistry recognizes the judicious use of lasers as a beneficial instrument in providing dental restorative and soft-tissue procedures for infants, children, and adolescents, including those with special health-care needs.

Studies indicate that general anesthesia may increase the risk for learning disabilities and behavioral problems such as attention-deficit/hyperactivity disorder (ADHD) in infants who are exposed to the anesthetic drugs several times.

Infants exposed to anesthesia were more than twice as likely to have a language disability. In particular, it increased the chance that a child would have trouble listening to and remembering spoken words.

Revising these tissues does not require placing the infant or child into the operating room under a general anesthesia.

The safety of dental lasers

The wavelength of the laser energy as well as the type of medium used to create the laser beam identifies lasers.

Unfortunately, there have been a few statements made by individuals unfamiliar with lasers that suggest that lasers are unsafe, that they can burn or cause blindness, or say that we revise and release frena to pay for our lasers. These rumors and misinformed statements are completely fabricated and have no scientific facts to support them.

I have used a variety of lasers, which include erbium, diodes, and carbon dioxide lasers since the year 2000 and have successfully revised or released more that ten thousand attachments as well as excised or incised other oral soft tissue lesions.

Today's lasers are not only used for soft tissue surgery but are also used for the removal of dental decay and to avoid the need for numbing.

Comments by patients

> As mother of three who had nursed well into toddlerhood, I knew something was amiss from the get-go with the birth of our fourth child. When she latched immediately after birth, I

was left with a blood blister on my nipple, and the pain was excruciating. Luckily my sister is an IBCLC and an RN, and she was able to help me figure out, through teleconferences and phone calls, that tongue-tie was likely the problem. By day four of life I'd already switched to pumping every three hours instead of nursing. After a lot of phone calls, I was able to get an appointment with oral surgery at the Children's Hospital of Philadelphia (CHOP), an excellent children's hospital located IN my town, but was dismayed to learn that the surgeon would only perform the laser surgery at six weeks of age, and only under anesthesia.

Considering I already had three kids at home and that I returned to work part time the day after I delivered, I was beyond exhausted by pumping every three hours. Luckily again, my sister gave me Dr. Kotlow's information, and I was able to get an appointment within a matter of days. Baby girl got the laser ablation done without anesthesia, on the day of the consultation. It was such a relief to be able to put her to the breast immediately after and nurse without pain and to offer her comfort. Moreover, Dr. Kotlow performed her lip-tie as well, which CHOP told us was purely cosmetic and that insurance would not pay for.

Dr. Kotlow's staff was incredibly helpful at accommodating our appointment in a timely manner and for helping us figure out our insurance coverage. The appointment ran incredibly smoothly and like clockwork. Dr. Kotlow showed us an informative video and gave us literature to read to prepare us for the wound care. Considering I'm a physician, and I know how challenging it can be to run on time, I was impressed by the friendliness of the staff and the timeliness of the appointment. I followed Dr. Kotlow's advice to follow up with a lactation consultant and see a craniosacral therapist, which helped me deal with those issues. They helped provide reassurance that we were on the right track. Nursing slowly improved over the following three weeks as my sore nipples healed, the baby's nursing technique improved and her wounds healed, and my oversupply was tamed.

Now that the baby is seven months, I can happily report that she is a portly twenty pounds and is thriving. Her reflux resolved with the oversupply issue, and she nurses easily. We followed *the instructions Dr. Kotlow gave us in regards to wound care and have not experienced any recurrence of her tongue- and lip-ties.*

I'd recommend Dr. Kotlow to any of my friends in a similar situation. Thank you, Dr. Kotlow!

Which lasers are ideal for treating infants?

Erbium lasers: There are primarily three types of lasers used by most dentists for infant soft-tissue surgery. The erbium family of lasers, which was originally developed for use in restoring decayed teeth and then was found to be successful in many soft-tissue procedures. The primary drawback with erbium lasers is that they are the least efficient in preventing bleeding.

Diode lasers: The second family of lasers is known collectively as diode lasers and represents lasers that have a variety of different wavelengths. The most efficient of these diode lasers is the XLase 1064 laser manufactured by Technology4dentistry.

These lasers can only be used for soft-tissue surgery and have an excellent ability to prevent bleeding, but they can be slow. They should be used in the pulse mode. They require being in contact with the tissue to allow for ablation and ablate tissue by a photothermal heating of the tissue. They are often the least expensive laser to purchase.

Carbon dioxide lasers: The third groups of lasers are known as carbon dioxide lasers and are available in two different wavelengths. One laser operates in the area of 10,600-nanometer wavelength and is only used for soft tissue surgery. The most recently developed and the present state-of-the-art laser is the isotopic carbon dioxide laser—manufactured by Convergent Dental and called the Solea laser—which operates in the area of 9,300 nanometers. This laser can be used to treat all hard- and soft-tissue dental procedures, and it is the fastest and easiest laser to use.

Laser safety and eye protection: Proper safe use of any dental laser requires that the operator be trained in the knowledge of laser physics and laser safety, and has hand-on training before going to a patient's mouth. Once these objectives are met, the laser surgeon can produce excellent results.

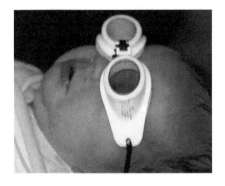

Laser goggles placed on an infant. Laser surgery requires that everyone, including the infant, have special laser glasses placed on his or her eyes when the laser is in use. Laser eye patches are also available but require the use of an adhesive and may cause soft tissue irritation. Laser goggles are available through innovativeoptic.com.

Controlling infant mobility during laser surgery

Achieving good stability of an infant requires the infant to be wrapped in a suitable restraining device such as a baby blanket or swaddling clothes (a sleeping bag-like pouch) or receiving blanket to control unwanted arm and leg movement. In the case of older infants a protective restraining appliance may also be required. This is the correct position for your assistant to hold the infant during the surgical revisions.

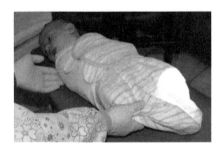

Most infants under the age of one year can easily and safely be treated and have their movements controlled by using a simple infant swaddler available in almost every baby clothing store.

Protecting your infant's airway during surgery

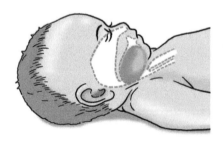

Poor head position with a closed airway

Successfully treating infants requires the right surgical skills, a knowledge of surgery, and a well-trained and knowledgeable staff. Positioning the infant for surgery requires that the infant's airway is protected and the head position is maintained so the airway does not get compromised. Positioning and stabilizing the infant is very important to achieving a successful release.

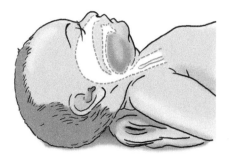 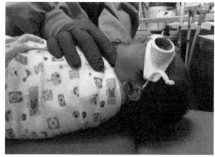

Infant placed in correct position maintaining an open airway.

Doing surgery in such small mouths

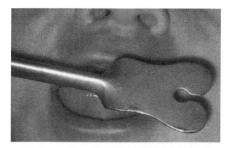

An instrument known as a grooved tongue director is used to elevate and control the tongue. This is especially helpful in infants with very small mouths and there is limited space for accessing the surgical area.

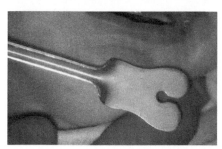

When using the grooved director, always make sure to hold the smooth side on the infant's skin area to prevent leaving an impression of the handle on the cheeks.

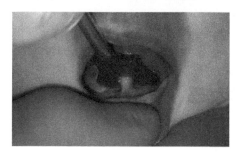

The grooved director is an instrument which will control the tongue movement and is especially helpful in newborns and infants who have small mouths which would make access difficult.

Isotopic carbon dioxide laser (*SOLEA Convergent Dental)

Once the infant is properly prepared for surgery, the laser of choice is used. The isotopic carbon dioxide laser can be placed outside the surgical area, since the laser beam is quite effective in releasing the tissue from a distance as much as 2–3 inches and can easily revise the smallest infant's tongue-tie. To release the tissue the laser-aiming beam is placed into the middle of the attachment and then the area is ablated leaving a clear, non-bleeding surgical site.

Isotopic carbon dioxide laser lingual attachment release

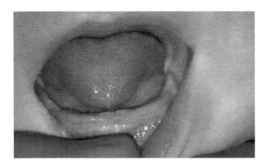

This infant displays a severe class IV tongue-tie attachment.

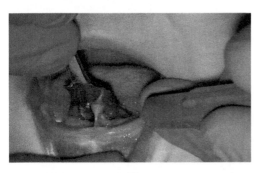

Initial location for the placement of the Solea CO2 laser in the center of the tongue frenum attachment.

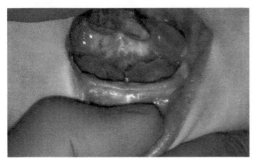

Immediate post surgical release of the tethered tongue attachment.

Isotopic carbon dioxide laser release of the upper lip-tie

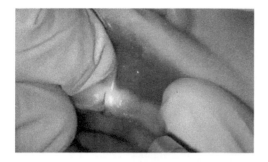

Initial placement of the Solea CO2 laser at the Class III insertion point of the maxillary lip-tie.

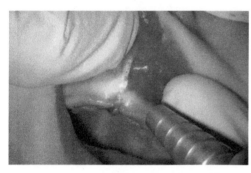

Initial ablation or removal of the tight frenum attachment.

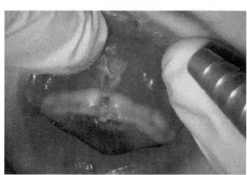

Immediate post surgical release allowing the lip total freedom to extend upward during infant latch.

Isotopic carbon dioxide laser release of a buccal tie

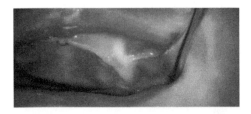

Upper buccal tie interfering with the infant's ability to achieve a good latch.

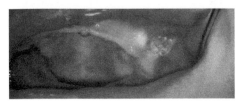

Immediate post surgical release of the tethered buccal frenum using the Solea CO_2 laser.

Diode laser revisions

There are many different wavelengths that can be identified as a diode laser. Having experienced using a variety of these lasers, I find the most effective one for a soft-tissue only laser to be the 1,064 diode (Xlase).

Release of tongue-tie using 1064 nm diode photothermal laser

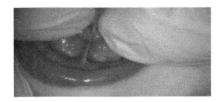

Presurgical attachment of the lingual attachment.

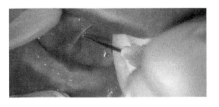

Placement of the Diode (XLase 1064 laser) laser in contact with the lingual frenum attachment.

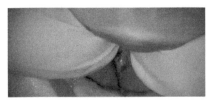

Post-surgical appearance after lingual frenum release using the 1064 diode laser.

Releasing the lip-tie using the 1064 diode

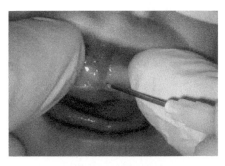

Pre-surgery appearance of the maxillary lip-tie.

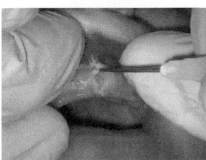

XLase Diode laser placement starting at insertion point of the maxillary lip-tie.

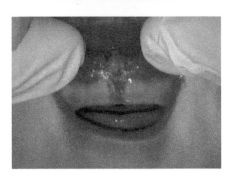

Post-surgical appearance after maxillary lip-tie frenum release using the 1064 diode laser.

CHAPTER 14

Post-surgical Active Wound Management

Having your infant's TOTs revised and not following up with the recommended post-surgery care will result in many of the surgeries rehealing back together. Preparing your infant for stretching activities will prevent both the parent and child from becoming upset.

Before beginning to stretching—post-surgery suck training

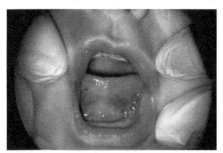

After surgery before any stretching begins, start initially with a gentle massage of the cheeks and lips externally until the infant opens his or her mouth. DO THIS AS WELL AT TIMES WHEN YOU ARE NOT STRETCHING THE SURGICAL SITES.

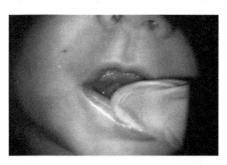

Introduce your fingers to the infant by slowly massaging the gum pads. Then slowly massage the roof of the mouth extending your index finger just forward of the junction of the hard and soft palate. Move the finger in a forward and backward motion maintaining contact with the hard palate tissue.

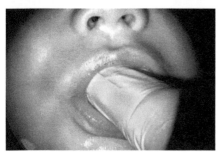

The infant's tongue should easily slip under your fingernail and allow for the gentle painless sucking action on the area between the fingers first two knuckles. This is also helpful when transitioning from the nipple shield to the breast skin.

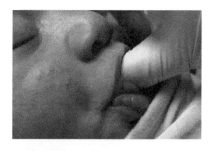

Post-surgery, if the infant appears to be uncomfortable, having him or her suck on your finger using breast milk or a little sugar water may help calm the infant.. Notice how the tongue now is able to slip under the finger. This is how the infant should latch when nursing—onto the areola, not the nipple.

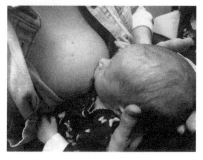

A one-month-old five-week-premature infant nursing on nipple shield immediately after surgical release of the lip and tongue tie. After surgery some infants will immediately go onto the breast and in others it may take up to a week to transition. Your IBCLC can assist in this transition if the problem continues.

Primary healing vs. secondary healing

Upon the completion of surgery eliminating the infant's restricted tissues, maintaining a successful surgery will be dependent on three things. Initially it is important to prevent the two sides of the surgical site from healing together to their original position by primary closure.

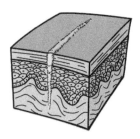

In primary healing, the two sides of an incision or cut heal together and attempt to re-create the original appearance of the tissues prior to being severed. This is how a cut on your finger or arm would heal.

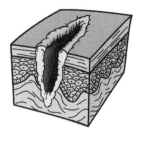

In revising an infant's attachments, the goal is to allow healing by allowing each area healing independently and separately, not returning to the prior appearance.

Active wound management requires that the surgical areas, both the lip and tongue, be repeatedly extended apart from each other for up to 2 weeks. Similar to my examination of your infant, **all post-surgery exercises must be done with the infant's head in your lap facing the same direction as your face.**

Post-surgery care of the upper lip requires an upward elevation; you must expose the entire surgical area as well as the inside of the upper lip. Your index fingers must either touch or almost touch each other when elevating the lip.

If you elevate the lateral borders of the lip only, you will not adequately open the surgical site, and the areas will most likely heal back together.

Post surgical management of the lingual surgical site

Two techniques for maintaining the lingual surgical site from primary attachment can be used. This is often the difficult and stressful part for parents and the source of surgical failure. It is imperative that the site is kept from healing back to its original position. This can only be accomplished when the two sites are kept separate.

Your ultimate goal is to peel the tongue away from the floor of the mouth. One way is to place the tongue blade directly into the middle of surgical site and pull the base of the tongue away from the floor of the mouth. The preferred and more efficient method requires parents to place two index fingers directly into the surgical area and firmly press down toward the floor of the mouth; at the same time, pull the tongue away from the area by pushing toward your feet and then peeling toward your stomach.

This exposes the entire lingual surgical site and keeps the areas from healing back together. If the stretching is only on the lateral border of the tongue, you will not achieve a good separation.

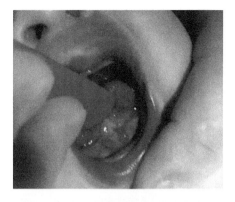

When using a tongue blade to keep the surgical areas apart use sufficient force to peel the tongue away from the floor of the mouth.

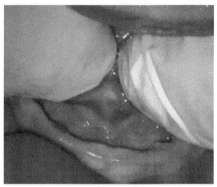

Placement of your index fingers at the base of the surgical area under the tongue to push downward on the floor of the mouth and peeling the tongue away, maintaining an open area.

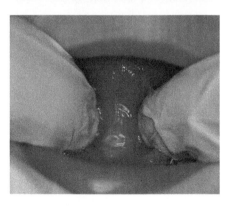

Appearance of a properly healing area under the tongue at 1 week.

Post-surgical active wound management is maintained three times a day, morning, afternoon and evening for two weeks. The surgical sites begin to turn white in most instances after one or two days. This is not any type of infection. It is a normal-appearing healing surgical site. Parents do not need to wear gloves, just wash hands.

Reopening and rehealing tongue attachment

If or when the areas under the tongue appear to be rehealing together, it is both necessary and possible to reopen the site easily by applying adequate force under the tongue to pop open the newly reformed frenum attachment.

If the tissue heals back together and you do need to reopen the surgical site, the area will most likely bleed. This is nothing to worry or be concerned about. Just calm your infant and place him or her directly onto the breast.

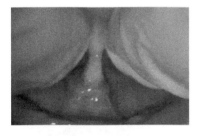

This is the appearance of the lingual frenum healing and forming a new attachment.

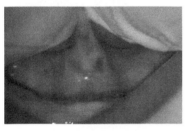

It is possible to reopen the area under the tongue in the first 3-4 weeks after surgery. Place your two index fingers at the base of the surgical area and firmly push down on the floor of the mouth until the area pops open.

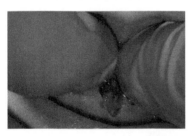

Appearance of the reopened lingual surgical area.

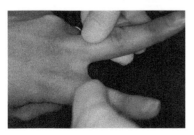

Correct pressure or force that needs to be placed on the tissue when stretching is approximately the same amount of pressure when stretching your fingers apart.

The following chart reviews this entire post-surgical process

Recommended post-surgical active wound management for new-born infants and toddlers after laser release of lingual-and upper lip-ties. Both surgical areas will turn white in a day or so. THIS IS NOT AN INFECTION BUT NORMAL HEALING TISSUE.

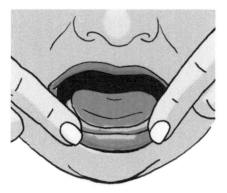

Your fingers in this position only allows elevation of the lateral borders of the tongue, this will not prevent the surgical sites from healing to their original position.

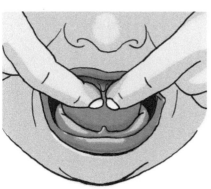

The correct way to prevent the tongue from healing back to the floor of the mouth is to place your index fingers on either side of the surgical site and push downward to the floor of the mouth and then sweep or peel the tongue away.

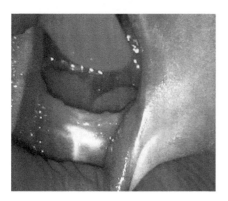

An alternative method is placing a tongue blade into the surgical site and pushing the tongue away from the floor of the mouth.

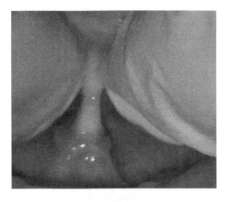

If the lingual frenum appears to be reforming, you need to use sufficient downward force to separate the two cut sites. You will then need to continue stretching for another week.

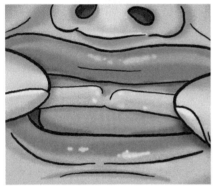

Just elevating the lateral borders of the upper lip when stretching to keep the surgical site open will result in the lip healing back together.

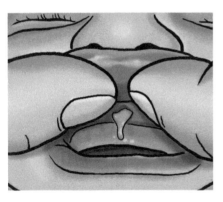

To prevent the upper lip-tie from healing back, you will need to elevate the lip upward exposing the entire inside of the upper lip as well as the entire surgical site. Failure to elevate the lip completely will result in partial healing of the surgical area together. Your index fingers should just touch. Gloved hands are not required when doing your post-surgery stretching. Just clean hands.

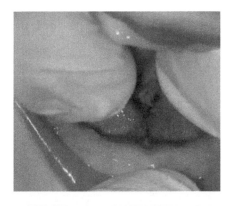

Gloved hands are not required when doing your post-surgery stretching. Just clean hands. To prevent the tongue and floor of the mouth from healing back together you need to first push downward into the floor of the mouth and then peel the tongue away towards your belly. Repeat this three times three times a day, morning, afternoon, and evening for two weeks.

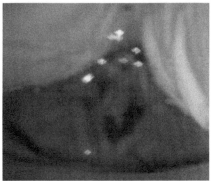

Some bleeding will most likely occur since the healing process requires the growth of new blood vessels into the healing areas. This will stop shortly or you can place the baby on the breast and this will also usually stop any bleeding.

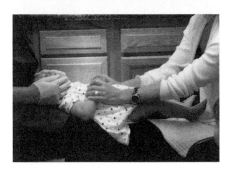

Require the infant to be placed with his or her head in your lap similarly to the way I examined and showed you the post-surgery care.

CHAPTER 15

The Other Members of the Breastfeeding Team Post-surgical Care

The post-surgery role of the IBCLC and bodyworker

My goal of successfully getting an infant a good seal and latch after the surgical release will also be dependent on post surgical care from your IBCLC and in some instances a pediatric chiropractor, osteopath, cranial-sacral therapist, or other experienced bodyworker.

Their goal will be to help you position your infants to achieve a proper latch and loosen tight head and neck muscles. Infants having long or traumatic births often are born with a condition called Torticollis, where your infant's neck may have been twisted during birth for a variety of reasons, which resulted in an asymmetrical head and neck position. Early intervention maximizes successful resolution of this problem and also assists in breastfeeding success.

Manual therapy involves a very gentle type of hands-on manipulation that is relaxing and is especially helpful for an infant's immature and developing neuromusculature system.

Infant therapy is a non-invasive treatment that helps relax your infant by reducing muscle stress and stiffness. Thus it aids the infant in achieving the full latching potential after the release of the tethered oral tissues. Manual therapy also reduces the crying and pain of the infant displaying signs of colic.

During the clinical evaluation of an infant, I routinely observe the condition of the cranial bone positions. I often see that the bones on the front top of the head may overlap slightly or that one side of the skull may be slightly elevated compared to the other side. During birth, the bones of the skull slide over each other so the infant can fit safely through the birth canal. After birth, the bones generally reposition themselves into the proper position, but sometimes they need gentle helping hands to accomplish this.

An infant's tongue should remain round when protruding. If the tongue appears pointy or heart-shaped when extended, this may indicate too much muscle tension. In cases where the tongue pulls to one side or another, this also interferes with the infant's ability to correctly latch the tongue during breastfeeding. For babies with more severe problems, the tongue may favor one side of the mouth while it is still completely within the oral cavity.

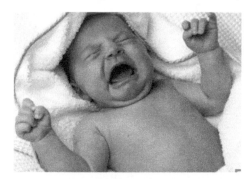

A tightly stressed infant. Crying, arms extended and body tight.

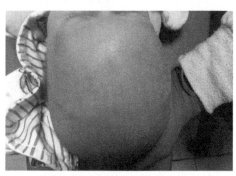

Overlapping of the cranial bones after delivery.

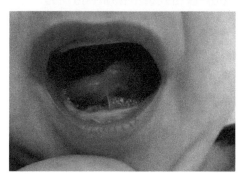

Pulling of the infants tongue to one side.

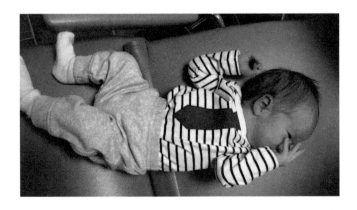

Infants undergoing long delivery stress, infants delivered by women with misaligned pelvic areas, or infants undergoing any other stressful encounter may deliver with significant body stress and will often appear to favor one side when resting. Bodyworkers can be extremely beneficial in reducing this misalignment to allow the infant to learn to attach to the breast more efficiently.

Body Fascia

Our entire body is incased by something known as fascia. Fascia is defined as a continuous, uninterrupted, three-dimensional, web-like tissue extending from our head to our toes, from the front to the back, interiorly to exteriorly. Fascia is connective tissue, which unites skin to the underlying tissues. It is found as facial membranes through out the body as well in our joint capsules, organ capsules, muscular coverings, ligaments, tendons, myo- and neurofascia, as well as other fibrous collagenous tissues. Since this includes connective tissues such as ligaments and fascia, the structure and alignment of the palate may also be influenced by the alignment of the other skull bones.

Techniques in manual medicine address the evaluation and diagnosis of structural dysfunction (a joint that does not move freely or in a full range of motion, a muscle that is short or lax, ligaments that have been injured, etc.). Structural dysfunction can simply cause a structural dysfunction—for example, if the joint between the jaw and the skull (tempromandibular joint) is misaligned because of manipulation at birth due to a prolonger or complicated labor.

Finally, when an infant is lying on his back, the baby should appear to lie with his body aligned in a straight line. Some babies turn and look like a C or take on a crescent-like appearance. If the infant is curved, when you gently straighten him out and he returns to that crescent position, the infant will benefit from attention from an appropriate practitioner.

Baby's hips and shoulders should appear level while he is resting. If you are working with a baby who is having trouble breastfeeding, and you see any of these postural symptoms, suggest to the mother that she consider taking her baby to a cranial-sacral therapist or pediatric chiropractor.

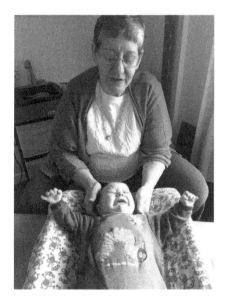
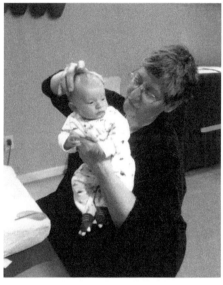

Pediatric Chiropractor Sharon Vallone treating infants both pre and post-lip and tongue-tie revisions to aid in completing the team effort to maximize the infant latch.

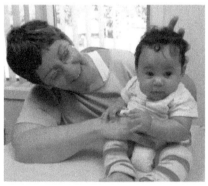

Comments by patients

As mother of three who had nursed well into toddlerhood, I knew something was amiss from the get-go with the birth of our fourth child. When she latched immediately after birth, I was left with a blood blister on my nipple, and the pain was excruciating. Luckily my sister is an IBCLC and RN, and she was able to help me figure out, through teleconferences and phone calls, that tongue-tie was likely the problem. By day four of life I'd already switched to pumping every three hours instead of nursing. After a lot of phone calls, I was able to get an appointment with an oral surgeon, but was dismayed to learn that the surgeon would only perform the laser surgery at six weeks of age, and only under anesthesia.

Considering I already had three kids at home and that I returned to work part-time the day after I delivered, I was beyond exhausted by pumping every three hours. Luckily again, my sister gave me Dr. Kotlow's information, and I was able to get an appointment within a matter of days. Baby girl got the laser ablation done without anesthesia, on the day of the consultation. It was such a relief to be able to put her to the breast immediately after and nurse without pain and to offer her comfort. Moreover, Dr. Kotlow released her lip-tie as well, which the surgeons told us was purely cosmetic and that insurance would not pay for.

Dr. Kotlow's staff was incredibly helpful at accommodating our appointment in a timely manner and for helping us figure out our insurance coverage. The appointment ran incredibly smoothly and like clockwork. Dr. Kotlow showed us an informative video and gave us literature to read to prepare us for the wound care. Considering I'm a physician and I know how challenging it can be to run on time, I was impressed by the friendliness of the staff and the timeliness of the appointment.

I followed Dr. Kotlow's advice to follow up with a lactation consultant and see a craniosacral therapist, which helped me deal with those issues. They helped provide reassurance that we were on the right track. Nursing slowly improved over the following three weeks as my sore nipples healed, the baby's nursing technique improved, and her wounds healed, and my oversupply was tamed.

Now that the baby is seven months, I can happily report that she is a portly twenty pounds and is thriving. Her reflux resolved with the oversupply issue, and she nurses easily. We followed the instructions Dr. Kotlow gave us in regard to wound care and have not experienced any recurrence of her tongue- and lip-ties.

Thank you, Dr. Kotlow!

CHAPTER 16

Air-Induced Reflux—Aerophagia

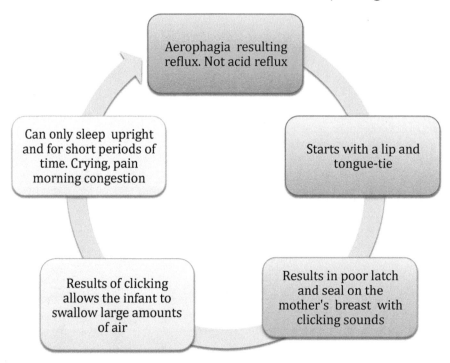

Reflux and Aerophagia

Physicians will often diagnose and treat infants with clinical signs of gastroesophageal reflux (GER) and in extreme cases gastroesophageal reflux disease (GERD). Infant reflux has classically been defined as a condition where the contents of the stomach are spit out, usually shortly after feeding.

A differential diagnosis of (GER) as well as its treatment can vary. It is sometimes recommended that the family wait it out, since the medical community feels that reflux in many instances will become less persistent as an infant gets older, or if the symptoms continue the reflux may be diagnosed as gastroesophageal reflux disease (GERD).

Although GER is not usually considered a pathological condition, its therapeutic management represents a controversial issue. Pharmacological treatment of GER may not resolve the issues.

The term gastroesophageal reflux (GER) is a diagnosis used commonly in preterm infants with these infants presenting with signs and symptoms of GER as high as 22%. Non-pharmacological approaches such as changing infant body positions or alternative feeding strategies may reduce or eliminate the problems.

GER is often attributed to an allergy or a blockage requiring surgical intervention when pyloric sphincter stenosis is present. Others suggest that spitting up and regurgitation are simply the usual symptoms of GER and that as long as an infant is healthy, content and growing well, the reflux and its symptoms are not a cause for concern or intervention. Comments such as your child will in all likelihood outgrow it are common.

Just wait it out and things get better in a few months

While it may be true that symptoms of (GER) will eventually resolve as the infant gets older, advising parents to just wait it out and have their infants continue to have pain, cry, act fussy, and remain uncomfortable from three to twelve months is not comforting for parents.

Infants spend a great amount of time lying in a supine or semi-supine position. This allows the movement of stomach's contents to move toward the esophagus, which in turn can cause GER symptoms to become more prevalent.

Infant nourishment in breastfed and bottle-fed infants is usually completely liquid for the first six months of life; thus the movement of the stomach's contents upward is even more probable and can contribute to the development of infant reflux symptoms.

Sometimes it is suggested that an infant might simply drink too much, too fast. Although infant reflux most often occurs after a feeding session, it can happen anytime an infant coughs, cries, or strains.

These diagnoses are made ignoring what is actually aerophagia-induced reflux (AIR).

Differential diagnosis

The common differential diagnosis for determining the causes of infant reflux include evaluation for such conditions as allergic gastroenteritis, which is defined as an intolerance to something in food, usually a protein in cow's milk.

Gastroesophageal reflux disease (GERD) is a more severe condition where the reflux is acidic enough to actually irritate and damage the lining of the esophagus. Eosinophilic esophagitis is an allergic condition where eosinophils infiltrate the lining of the esophagus.

A search of the existing literature indicates that in the vast majority of cases, TOTS is not considered in the evaluation of infants presenting with GER. When an infant is found to be swallowing large amounts of air into the stomach, a condition known as aerophagia or air-induced reflux, can force the stomach's content upward, which is then followed by regurgitation or even projectile vomiting of the contents. Health-care professionals usually disregard the effects of breastfeeding and how this can affect infant reflux.

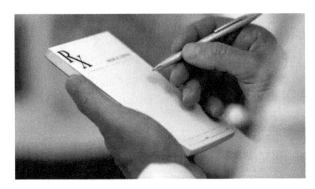

The initial rush to use drugs is neither beneficial nor recommended. Treatment of infant gastroesophageal reflux (GER) is to prescribe adult anti-reflux drugs. Infants are placed on oral medication: acid-blocking drugs like an H-2 blocker such as ranitidine (Zantac), a proton pump inhibitor such as omeprazole (Prilosec), or lansoprazole (Prevacid).

Pharmacologic treatment of infants with reflux symptoms is problematic. There appears to be little evidence to suggest that pharmacologic agents help these infants. Children taking these medications may also face an increased risk of certain intestinal and respiratory infections. In infants, prolonged use of proton pump inhibitors has been linked to problems in iron and calcium absorption.

Pharmacologic Management:

Gastroesophageal reflux (GER) occurs when the stomach contents flow back up into the esophagus of infants, and this often results in repeated episodes of projectile vomiting or regurgitation of the stomach's contents immediately after nursing. The involvement of ankyloglossia (tongue-tie) and upper lip-ties (TOTS) should be part of the differential diagnosis.

Adding evaluation of lip and tongue-ties to the differential diagnosis

Revising tethered oral tissues eliminates the need for any pharmacologic intervention, radiation, general anesthesia, hospitalization, blood tests, or other invasive procedure. In reality the correlation between lip-ties and tongue-ties and swallowing of air by infants is quite significant and needs to be part of any infant evaluation when reflux is suspected.

If physicians were to include these as part of their differential diagnoses many infants would be spared the need for these extensive tests and unnecessary drugs.

Infant symptom history

1. Vomiting after breastfeeding (also may occur with bottle-feeding)
2. The infant is unable to sleep while lying down
3. Constant irritability and crying unless held upright
4. Can only be comforted when sleeping in a parent's arms, infant car seat or a swing
5. The Infant wakes up congested in the morning, sometimes leading to treating the problem as an allergy to mother's milk
6. A physical history exam by the parents after nursing indicates the infant having a distended or hard belly after breastfeeding
7. A history of being very gassy
8. Evaluation of the mother's latch shows that the attachment to the mother's breast is weak, inconsistent, poor, and is associated with clicking or sucking in air into the stomach known as aerophasia. Aerophagia is a condition of excessive air swallowing, which goes to the stomach

9. Infants may have slow weight gain or a diagnosis of failure to thrive

10. Waking up congested every morning

Example of a patient with a laser release of the lip- and tongue-tie and a diagnosis of GERD

The following photos are from an eight-and-a-half-month-old infant who underwent all of the medical differential diagnostic procedures and genetic testing. The parents were told the infant might have severe developmental problems. **Revision of the lip and tongue resolved these problems.**

It is important to include tethered oral tissues such as tongue-ties and lip-ties as part of a differential diagnosis when an infant presents with signs of infant reflux. If it is found that these tissues restrict the infant from achieving a good latch, and they allow for ingestion of large amounts of air into the infant's belly, the tissue should be revised before more invasive procedures or the use of drugs to control the reflux are considered.

Clinical examination revealed the following:

This infant was seen at eight months of age and had the above-listed symptoms during the first eight months. The breastfeeding history included all of the prior symptoms. Delayed growth both physically and neurologically, use of a variety of different pharmacologic medications, hospitalizations, and tests to rule out Crohn's disease, celiac disease, genetic abnormalities.

Clinical evaluation of the lingual- and maxillary lip-ties indicated they were significantly tethered.

Post-surgical results as reported by the infant's mother:

The infant immediately latched the evening after revision; symptoms slowly resolved and by twelve months of age, the child was normal physically and neurologically.

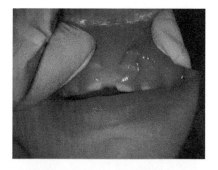

Preoperative photo of maxillary lip-tie: The presurgical appearance of the maxillary lip-tie indicated the existence of a wide diastema due to a thick, fibrous frenum attachment. The attachment interfered with the upper lip from flanging upward thus causing a shallow latch and preventing the infant from achieving a tight latch.

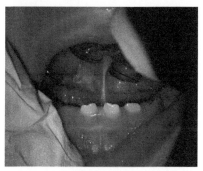

The presurgical appearance of the infant's tongue attachment to the floor of the mouth indicated the tongue was unable to extend forward, upward, or laterally, thus limiting the tongue's ability to express milk efficiently from the mother's breast.

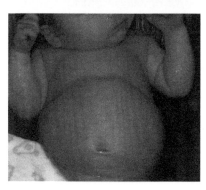

A photo of the infant after attempting to breastfeed shows the infant's belly distended with air due to the shallow latch and ingestion of air (aerophagia).

CHAPTER 17

Sleep Apnea

Infant sleep apnea can be a significant concern and may be caused when your infant's tongue is tethered and the tongue's resting position ends up in the infant's airway. This is often why an infant begins to gag whenever you place something such as a breast, a pacifier or a bottle into the infant's mouth. In effect you are blocking his or her airway.

This will also account for infants breaking their latch as soon as they begin to nurse. If the airway is blocked when the infant is sleeping on his or her backside, there is a potential for reduced oxygen flow to the brain and this can be a significant problem since during the early weeks the infant's brain and nervous system are growing at a rapid rate. Proper sleep and breathing determine health and development for the rest of an infant's life.

An infant sleeping with his or her mouth open, snoring or breathing with distress is something that needs to be fully evaluated. During an obstructive hypopnea, in comparison to an obstructive apnea, the airway is only partially closed.

Chronic airway-dependent breathing may be the stimulus to cause regrowth of tonsil or adenoidal tissues.

Obstructive sleep apnea (OSA) in infants should be a significant concern for both the parents and health-care professionals. The results of OSA may express themselves as cognitive impairment, attention and hyperactivity disorders, poor academic achievement, disruptive behavior in school and cardiovascular and metabolic complications.

In many instances once the tethered tongue is released these symptoms will disappear.

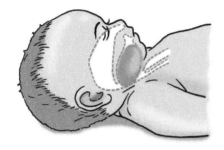 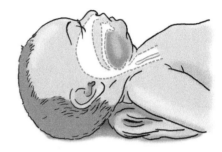

Infants and adults who have difficulty in maintaining an open airway when resting will suffer from obstructive sleep apnea.

An open airway allows for normal nasal breathing.

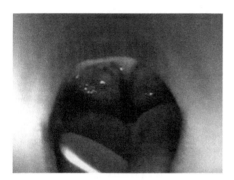

Enlarged tonsils or adenoids may contribute to dangerous mouth breathing. Ankyloglossia, or tongue-ties, should also be evaluated and treated when the airway is being obstructed.

Evaluating your infant for abnormal sleeping symptoms

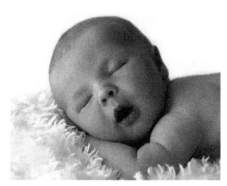

1. Pause between breathes that last 10–20 seconds or longer
2. Gasping for a breath
3. "Cute" snoring
4. Gagging
5. Face or body turning blue
6. Limp body
7. Slow heartbeat

Observing your infant's clinical symptoms

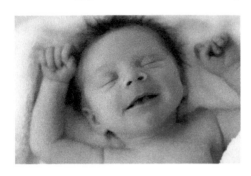

1. Lips apart—open mouth—
   Mouth breathing
2. Lateral borders of the tongue
   turned upward
3. Crease down center of the tongue
4. Tongue is not extending outward
5. Heart-shaped anterior border
6. Unable to elevate upward
7. Placing breast, pacifier, or bottle
   into mouth causes the infant to
   pull away
8. Compensatory breastfeeding
9. Self-weaning early
10. Adversarial mother-infant relation-
    ship that can last a lifetime!

Clinical airway obstruction concerns for toddlers and older children

A dental examination is not just about teeth, it is an examination of your child's entire oral health, head, and neck structures as they relate to oral structures, because all of these can affect your child's overall growth and development.

One part of an evaluation is examining your child's tonsils and visible upper airway for any abnormalities or problems.

The dentist should always be concerned with the upper airway and how it can affect oral shape and development of the upper and lower jaws. Medical science is also now becoming keenly aware that there is more to upper airway problems than just the development of the "long face" and malocclusions.

The diagnosis of asthma has been used many times when infants and young children are having breathing difficulties, children can be labeled as ADHD or ADD, and mental development can be effected when sleep apnea prevents adequate oxygen to reach your child's brain, in some instances reducing the IQ by as much as ten points.

Snoring is not cute. It represents a blocked airway.

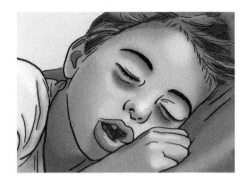

Many parents think, when they peek in and listen to their infant sleeping and hear a snoring infant that it is cute. In fact, this is an indication that the airway is in some way being obstructed and may be a sign of future problems.

The following are the most common symptoms of obstructive sleep apnea. However, every child is different and symptoms may vary. Symptoms may include:

_____**Noisy breathing** during daytime or sleep

_____**Snoring**—any snoring or noisy breathing during sleep. (Perception is occasional snoring is okay)

_____**Periods of not breathing**—although the chest wall is moving, no air or oxygen is moving through the nose or mouth into the lungs. The duration of these periods is variable and measured in seconds.

_____**Mouth breathing**—the passage to the nose may be completely blocked by enlarged tonsils and adenoids leading to the child only being able to breathe through his/her mouth.

_____**Bloated bellies**—due to aerophagia (swallowing large amounts of air)

_____**Restlessness during sleep**—the frequent arousals lead to restless sleeping or "tossing and turning" throughout the night.

_____**Sleeping in odd positions**—the child may arch his neck backward (hyperextend) in order to open the airway or sleep sitting up.

_____**Behavior problems or sleepiness**—may include irritability, crankiness, frustration, hyperactivity, and difficulty paying attention.

_____**School problems**—children may do poorly in school, even being labeled as "slow" or "lazy."

_____**Bed wetting**—also known as nocturnal enuresis, although there are many causes for bedwetting besides sleep apnea.

_____**Frequent infections**—may include a history of chronic problems with tonsils, adenoids, and/or ear infections.

_____**Allergies**—diagnosed with suspected allergies that may be due to restricted airways and breathing

If a child has any of the above symptoms and a clinical appearance of airway blockage while being examined lying down, I recommend that you see a qualified ENT physician to evaluate your child's tonsils and adenoids as well as a possible sleep study to determine if he or she has obstructive sleep apnea, sleep-disruptive disease, or sleep disorder symptoms. This problem is serious and may affect your child for a lifetime if not evaluated and if need be, corrected early.

CHAPTER 18

What Are the Potential Problems if Parents choose not to revise the TOTs?

Parents often go back to their primary-care physician and ask his or her opinion about revisions or release of the upper lip-tie or lingual attachment. Unfortunately, since this is really a dental question, and not a medical one, the information they receive is often both incomplete and just plain wrong. Some of the effects of doing nothing may include some or all of the following:

The night time tooth-brushing fights!

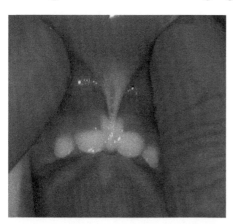

The upper frenum or lip –tie in this patient created undue stress. Whenever the parent tried to brush the upper front teeth by elevating the lip to gain access to the upper front teeth caused discomfort and actually was starting to slightly tear the tissue. The frenum would blanch and pull when elevated. Release of the tie eliminated all the discomfort, as well made tooth-brushing a comfortable bedtime experience.

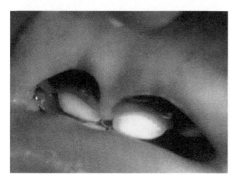

Infants presenting with this appearance of the lip-tie, especially after a fall have been known to be seen in the hospital emergency room where the lip was thought to be stuck between the two front teeth.

Intercepting potential malocclusion: avoiding the diastema

The class III and Class IV lip-tie may interfere with the eruption of the primary upper central incisors.

This can carry forward to the upper permanent teeth as well. Depending on the size and shape of the lip-tie tissue, the gap size can vary.

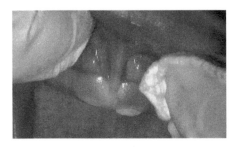

Infant just beginning to erupt upper front teeth with diastema or gap forming.

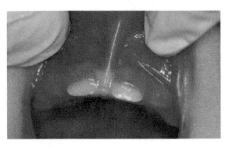

Upper front teeth erupting with large diastema or gap.

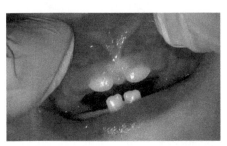

Upper front teeth erupted with facial decay beginning.

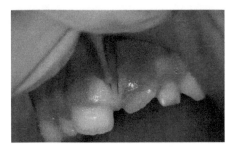

Permanent teeth erupting and being pushed laterally due to the lip-tie.

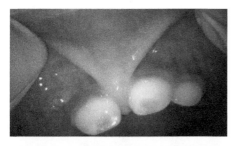

Initial stages of facial decay.

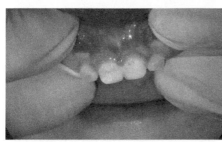

Decay beginning to involve four front teeth.

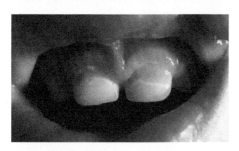

Deep, extensive decay occurring.

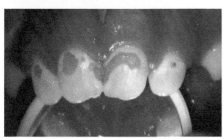

Fully involved upper front teeth on infant at-will nursing with lip-tie.

As discussed earlier in this book, when mothers choose to at-will breastfeed during the night after the eruption of the primary upper incisors, the milk can become trapped in the folds of the tightly tethered lip and allow the formation of facial decay. Different degrees of decay can be created depending on the length of time the milk remains in contact with the facial surfaces of these teeth.

The untreated tongue-tie: the beginning of oral dysfunction

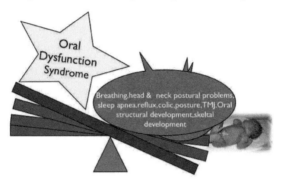

When a diagnosis of the tethered tongue is made, not releasing the tongue can often begin a cascading series of problems we can list as oral dysfunction. As the above graphic describes from the beginning of allowing the tongue's mobility to be impaired eventually interferes with a variety of respiratory, skeletal, neuromuscular, GI, and in the future, potential cardiac problems. When any or all of these problems occur they can have a devastating effect on the individual's psychological and self-image development.

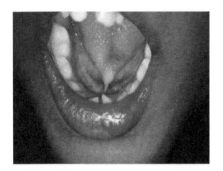

If the lingual frenum is very tight it may be contributing to the formation of a malocclusion. These two photos show the lower central incisors being displaced lingually. If this persists in the adult dentition over time it will pull the gum tissue away from the lower front teeth causing periodontal disease, it also interfere with any future orthodontic care.

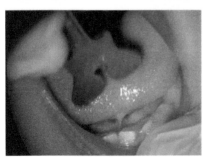

The malocclusion begins as soon as the eruption of the first lower primary teeth. Lower front teeth being pulled lingually.

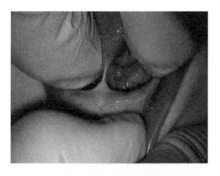

This total class IV attachment restricts the tongue function, leading to potential speech articulation problems, sleep apnea, and chewing and swallowing solid foods, and it can affect the development of the maxillary arch, leading to a high arched palate and a malocclusion.

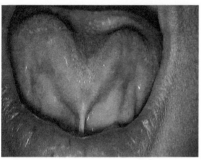

In adult dentition, this can affect breathing, be a contributing factor in sleep apnea, affect sexual activity, contribute to TMJ disease, and allow for the development of shoulder, head, and neck pain.

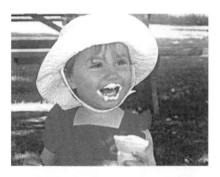

One of the things we all enjoy is eating. When the tongue is tethered and cannot function correctly, it may interfere with the normal movements of the tongue required to chew and move food through the mouth, and the natural cleaning of our teeth. The act of just eating an ice-cream cone can be difficult and messy as well as embarrassing.

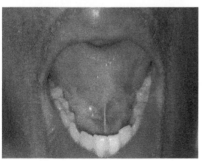

The tongue-tie in this adult patient affected the lateralization of the mandibular jaw and position of the posterior teeth, and the constricted lower jaw.

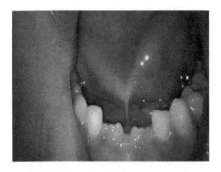

The tight lingual attachment prevents the lower anterior teeth from migrating together. The lower diastema will be created.

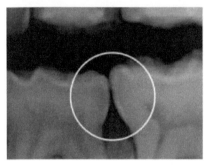

The inability of the tongue to act as a toothbrush and help remove food particles, especially in the lower jaw, can result in extensive tooth decay in the areas on the biting surface as well as the areas between the molars.

CHAPTER 19

What to Expect After Surgery

Nursing strike for 24 hours

After the surgical release or revisions of the lingual, labial, or other TOTs have been completed, infants may latch immediately. Others may latch immediately while still in my office, and then go on a strike for 24–48 hours. In rare instances, it may take a week for some babies to become good breastfeeding infants.

Nipple shields

Mothers who arrive requiring a nipple shield to achieve a good latch will sometimes achieve a good skin-to-skin attachment after a few minutes and others may take a week to transition from plastic to skin.

Post-surgery discomfort

Discomfort is also a variable. Post-surgical discomfort will often depend on the type of attachment that was revised. A thick wide surgical site will be more likely to cause discomfort for 24–48 hours than release of a very thin membrane.

Post-surgical active wound management will also be dependent on the degree of surgical release required.

Rewiring the infant's brain

Infant's brains are wired from birth to breastfeed as soon as they are born. When babies are prevented from achieving an effective latch their brains will attempt to compensate for this and the longer this compensation occurs, the longer it will take for them to relearn what the brain originally wanted to achieve. Some infants learn quickly and some take time.

Pacifiers

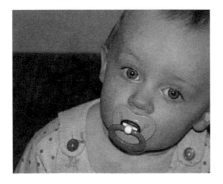

Many parents ask about using a pacifier. The pacifier acts as a replacement for the breast when the breastfeeding is non-nutritional. After revision, you may be able to reduce the use. Using a pacifier after surgery is okay. However, the use of pacifiers in general can lead to significant orthodontic problems.

Understanding this is a team effort

The learning process often requires the team effort by the surgeon, the IBCLC, and the bodyworker. Skipping any one of these steps often results in premature weaning. This early weaning is often associated with maternal depression due to the failure to achieve the type of bond the mother anticipated in the months prior to delivery.

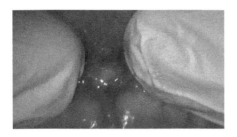

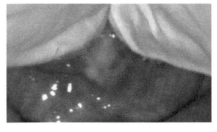

The upper lip-tie will begin to turn white in a day or so. This is normal. Infections do not happen after these surgical procedures and are not a complication or concern. The diamond in the surgical site will eventually be replaced by normal appearing tissue. Infants who are not mobile will rarely have bleeding, older infants who could poke or hit the area while moving may create some bleeding. If bleeding does appear, a moist non-verbal tea bag placed at the surgical site will stop the bleeding in a few minutes.

The area under the tongue will also turn white to yellow after a few days, and this is not an infection. If you see any red around the surgical site, it is nothing to be concerned about—just normal healing. If the center of the cut has a red line or bleeding, it means you have reopened the area that was beginning to heal back together.

Homeopathic remedies

If infants appear to be in distress after surgery, over-the-counter homeopathic remedies, such as Rescue Remedy, can be safely used. Finger-sucking exercises with mother's milk or small amounts of a dilute solution of sugar water also help calm the crying infant.

CHAPTER 20

Myofunctional Therapy

For patients with tethered oral tissues, myofunctional therapy is also often important in obtaining a complete recovery of the restricted oral tissues. This may prevent or possibly avoid relapse or revision in the future. For infants, stretching, stroking and massaging are all necessary. The motion of breastfeeding becomes easier and can be used as therapy for both parent and child. Bodywork such as cranial osteopathy, cranial chiropractic work and cranial-sacral therapy is essential to the unwinding and normalizing of the entire body functions.

Myofunctional therapy is the neurologic re-education of the oral facial muscles. It is a therapy program designed to re-pattern chewing, swallowing and breathing through the use of therapeutic techniques and positive behavioral modification. Therapy allows the brain to develop new neuro-pathways to the muscles through repetition and time, which is known as neuroplasticity.

When the revisions of TOTS are performed, the body needs to allow for healing while integrating a new pattern of muscle functions. OMT facilitates the body's healing process which may help to prevent scar tissue from developing or reattachment. For the treatment of children and adults with TOTs, therapy should begin at least one month prior to the release and then followed for at least 8 -11 months after procedure.

Myofunctional therapy is also recognized as an important modality in the treatment of temporomandibular jaw dysfunction (TMJ), chronic headaches, malocclusion, drooling, functional posture problems, some digestive disorders, and some ear problems.

This therapy can also help eliminate oral habits such as mouth breathing, thumb sucking, nail, lip, hair or object chewing, which may interfere with proper growth and development of the mouth and face. The tongue needs to be re-trained to replace the habit. The treatment may also help to prevent some orthodontic problems and gum disease.

By normalizing the orofacial functions with myofunctional therapy, these disorders may dissipate. By establishing nasal breathing as the norm, many problems with allergies, sleep apnea, sinus infections and middle ear problems may diminish.

We now have evidence-based research (more than 300 studies) to consider myofunctional therapy as an adjunctive treatment of obstructive sleep apnea in both adults and children. Because so many of the symptoms of sleep disorders involve the functions of the tongue and breathing, myofunctional therapy may be a first line defense in not only the early intervention of sleep apnea but also for the ongoing treatment and prevention of this disorder.

Additionally, myofunctional therapy is a therapeutic program by which articulation problems are often improved because the patients have better control of their muscle functions and tongue placement.

The treatment also offers an aesthetic benefit. By improving the function of the facial muscles, a more relaxed, natural, defined facial appearance may develop. Many times the patients self esteem may improve.

Furthermore, because the tongue is attached to the hyoid bone in the neck, this method enables recipients to learn beneficial patterns, which may improve head and neck postures and chronic neck or back pain.

This form of treatment may be used by dental hygienists, speech pathologists, physical therapists, occupational therapists, physicians, dentists or other allied health professionals who have completed a post graduate training course in myofunctional therapy.

For more information on myofunctional therapy

The Academy of Orofacial Myofunctional Therapy (AOMTinfo.org) and the Academy of Applied Myofunctional Sciences. (AAMSinfo.org)

CHAPTER 21

The Orthopostural Factor

The first few weeks of life are crucial as the baby transitions from its safe and comfortable watery home into the big wide world, where it has to cope with so many different conditions and situations.

Whatever we can do, as parents or therapists, to make this transition as smooth as possible, will greatly affect the peace, happiness and correct growth of the baby.

The word ortho-postural literally means <u>straight posture</u>, and that refers to various parts of the body, not only the way we stand.

In the infant, the posture of the tongue, the head and the neck is critical to being able to nurse effectively, and if it is compromised in any way, several dysfunctions can occur which can cause lifelong issues.

Very few people are aware of several unique properties of the tongue.

- It is not a muscle – it is a group of 8 different muscles all working in harmony. 4 are internal, are not attached to any bone, and change the shape of the tongue. The other 4 are external, are in pairs, are attached to bone, and are responsible for the position of the tongue.

- It is, gram for gram, one of the strongest 'muscles' in the body.

- It is the only 'muscle' in the body that is attached at one end only - every other muscle has two points of attachment. The tongue cannot function unless it first 'grounds' itself.

- Ideally, it should do this by pressing against the upper jaw, behind where the front teeth will be, and when in this position it rises up against the palate, forming a 'bump' which pushes liquids and solids down into the esophagus. This movement should be almost imperceptible, and if you see movement of the muscles of the lips and cheeks, you can be sure that the swallowing pattern is dysfunctional.

- It has a rich blood and nerve supply and is so sensitive that even something as small as a hair can be easily felt.

What can go wrong?

- The major issue with tongue function is whether it is tied or tethered, meaning it is not able to move freely within the mouth.

- The first thing that this does is to interfere with latching – so nursing becomes very difficult and frustrating.

- If the baby cannot move the tongue freely it will swallow air, bite and push in order to express the milk, and this can be a very painful process – as well as being a traumatic experience for both Mom and baby

Tongue and lip ties can often be related to the Mom's health, nutrition, stress levels and general health condition during the stage when the tongue and lips were being formed.

Other feeding, suckling and swallowing problems can come from:

- the way the baby was lying in the womb
- the birth process
- cranial strains
- traumatic interventions such as
  - o C-Section
  - o Vacuum extraction
  - o Forceps delivery

It is such a simple process to have a baby checked at birth – yet so many doctors and pediatricians do not take these important steps.

In these modern times, where we are stressed, overfed and undernourished, where we are surrounded by electromagnetic waves at every turn, and have environmental toxins all around us, there is the potential for our developing babies to develop compromises which could turn into chronic problems later in life.

Every baby born should be checked by an experienced and competent neonatal cranial therapist to make sure that:

- all 22 bones of the head are in the right place

- tongue and lips are free to latch and suckle

- there is no unnatural turning or twisting of the head and neck

These simple checks and interventions can make the difference between a baby that blossoms and thrives, rather than one that struggles and battles to overcome issues which could have been detected right at the start.

The greatest gift we can give our children is the best possible start in life.

OPTIMAL INFANT CARE IS NOT *OPTIONAL* INFANT CARE

Roger L. Price B.Sc. Hons. Pharm. D,
Consultant Respiratory Physiologist
Functional Medicine Educator.

CHAPTER 22

Conclusion

My goal in writing this book is to help mothers and fathers find the answer as to why their lives have been turned upside down with the birth of their infant. Many healthcare professionals with whom they depend on and seek out for answers and help do not provide answers and worse can be met with indifference.

It is also a book to be read as well by IBCLCs, midwives, nurses, hygienists, physicians, dentists, and others who deal with breastfeeding infants.

Unfortunately the stories that are contained within this book are all too real and continue to affect these families. My intent and hope is to help resolve these issues and get families appropriate care.

Infants and mothers experiencing difficulties with breastfeeding, primarily due to an ineffective or poor latch, experience many symptoms. Breastfeeding involves two individuals, the mother and the infant, and if either one of these individuals suffer symptoms related to an infant's latch, then revising both of these areas will usually improve the breastfeeding experience.

Is this whole issue just a passing fad?

Questions often arise about revising tethered tissues. Is it just a fad, or is it a real problem. Why does it seem there are more infants undergoing these revisions?

The answer is simple and to the point.

Today there are many more women choosing to breastfeed. The percentages are almost 90% of women in the United States in 2015 compared to around 20% in the early 1970s. Thus with more women breastfeeding, more mothers will show symptoms and require assistance. Too many examinations are completed while the infant rests in the mother's lap and this results in missing many of the lingual ties.

Breastfeeding should be a time where mothers and infants bond. This is best accomplished when breastfeeding is pleasurable and comfortable.

Breastfeeding should not be painful and challenging.

Breastfeeding should be a time when mothers, fathers, and infants bond together.

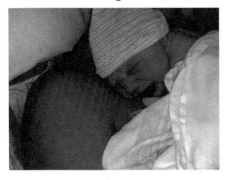 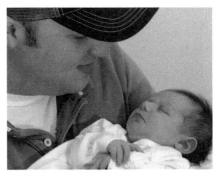

Infant bonding begins immediately after birth for the mother and infant. All too often, fathers are forgotten, but they are also part of the bonding experience. When mothers and infants suffer from breastfeeding difficulties, it will affect the father equally.

"We as healthcare professionals have a great capacity for choice and to make change. To make these important changes

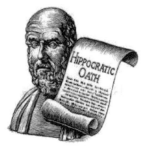

The medical and dental community needs to come together and realize what the Hippocratic Oath states: *"I will prescribe a regimen for the good of my patients according to my ability and judgment and never do no harm to anyone."* Allowing parents to suffer needlessly when a simple, safe, in-office procedure can effectively alleviate these problems, *does not fulfill this oath.*

we need to address the immovable attitudes of the unwilling, usually led by individuals that are unknowing, who dig in their heels and resist doing what is sensible for our infants and parents. Many of us have done so much, for so long, with so little support from the medical community. However, we are now more qualified to do so much for our patients. We are providing life support for families, infants, mothers and fathers when others are failing them."

Dr. Kotlow

Comments by patients

Dr. Kotlow was a dream come true for my son and my family. Sadly we found out really late (my son is two) that he was lip-tied. His severe upper lip-tie was either missed or ignored by every health-care professional to date, including two nursing coaches at the hospital. In my opinion all nurses who are coaching or helping women to nurse should be educated in the field of both upper and lower lip/tongue-ties. I had painful nursing and eventually had to give up and manually express my milk for eight months till my supply ran out. I diagnosed my son's upper lip-tie myself after being ignored by his primary care provider who merely provided excuse after excuse for trouble nursing, delayed speech, and decaying upper front teeth. I was told he would nurse better as he got older. I was told that it would just become less painful over time. Ladies, nursing should NOT be painful. I was told his speech was delayed because he's a boy, and boys simply talk later than girls. I was told the brown tint on his front four teeth was from sippy cups and juice and pacifier use. None, I repeat, NONE of these brush-offs were true. My son had upper lip-tie. The brittle decaying teeth were from breast milk and other food and drink being stuck between his upper lip and upper teeth creating a breeding area for bacteria.

Had I not been so lucky as to stumble across a Facebook post mentioning lip-ties and nursing pain, I would have never found out my son had a lip-tie and subsequently found Dr. Kotlow. We drove six hours to Dr. Kotlow's office for his frenectomy and I would do it again in a hear beat! I swear the waiting room was designed for my son! He was entertained the entire wait. With a motion-activated floor mat and interactive train station, it was a little toddler's dream. My son was very comfortable with Dr. Kotlow, and they always say children are the best judges of character. He allowed Dr. Kotlow to look in his mouth without much resistance at all. He allowed Dr. Kotlow to give him the sedation medication without any issue whatsoever. My son, even while waiting the hour for the medication to take effect, continually asked for the doctor. He had taken a liking to him and that eased a lot of fears for me.

My son, because of all previous inferior medical care required four porcelain veneers on his upper front teeth—hence the se-

dation. I was nervous, but I had no reason to be. My son wasn't even scared. He gladly went to the doctor when the time was right and returned with pretty uplifted spirits and in minimal pain. I have a very sensitive boy and had he been scared or in pain, he wouldn't have been shy to show it. Once the doctor mentioned ice cream, he was all ready to go! Dr. Kotlow really took to our story and was very social and informative. He was smart and kind, and these may not be attributes most look for in a doctor, but I don't like to feel like herded cattle in any doctor's office. Dr. Kotlow really made us feel like we mattered and that he cared for us and our child. He provided me with all the papers needed for care and even told me to text him if we needed anything.

Thank you so much, Dr. Kotlow for taking such great care of my son. For providing excellent dental care. For saving my son's teeth. For almost INSTANTLY improving his speech. It's only been one week and already my son is finding his voice! His words are more clear, and he's isn't struggling to express thoughts. I think he had all but given up on speaking because of the upper lip-tie. Once the frenectomy was done, it was as though everything came to him. He went from barely saying two words together which were not clear or crisp, to now putting entire phrases of words together and talking up a storm! Dr. Kotlow, you are a blessing to our family.

*   *   *

Almost six months ago I brought my son in to fix his tongue-and lip-tie. I was so concerned about the pain he'd be in that I delayed getting it done. My son was back in my arms and nursing within ten minutes. I figured he was in too much pain to really latch on because it didn't hurt! I was thrilled to find out that breastfeeding doesn't have to hurt and can be really enjoyable. I was shocked and overjoyed that he instantly had a better latch and I had no more pain. After three cases of mastitis and a breast abscess from his poor latch, I never thought we'd have such a great breastfeeding relationship. Our only regret is that we did not do it sooner. We are so fortunate to have Dr. Kotlow in the capital region. Don't be scared to go for a consult as your child could not be in better hands.

After we discovered our two-month-old was beginning to lose weight, we made the two-hour trip to Dr. Kotlow's office (they got us in the same week). Turns out our daughter was stage-four 100% tongue- and lip-tied. The surgery took no longer than five minutes and she was back in our arms. After a few days, she was eating better then ever and has now gained almost a pound in less then two weeks! We couldn't be happier and thank Dr. Kotlow and his staff for helping our little girl.

* * *

My daughter had colic and has had issues with reflux since the day she was born. I tried to breastfeed, and she would not latch even when using a guard. Her doctor immediately put her on formula for colic and Zantac for reflux. Now six and a half months later I just happened to be looking in her mouth to see if any teeth were coming in and I noticed that her top lip didn't look right. I found Dr. Kotlow's website, and after looking at pictures, I realized she had a maxillary lip tie. I immediately called Dr. Kotlow, as the more I researched online, the more information and stories I heard about what an amazing job he does. While on the phone with him, he told me how to check if she was also tongue-tied and she was. She was scheduled to go see a gastroenterologist to find out what was causing her to constantly vomit. I canceled that appointment as soon as Dr. Kotlow told me that the maxillary lip-tie and tongue-tie will cause colic and reflux. My daughter just had the procedure done by Dr. Kotlow three days ago, and she is already off the Zantac and doing amazing. I wish I had found Dr. Kotlow in the beginning as her lip- and tongue-tie had gone unnoticed by two doctors for six and a half months. I tried countless bottles, holding her upright for an hour after every feeding, and went through fifteen bibs a day, not to mention how it has affected her. I cannot thank Dr. Kotlow enough, and I highly recommend him. "

* * *

I want to share my experience with any mother considering Dr. Kotlow for a lingual frenectomy. I went to four dentists who were known to do frenectomies in Chicago. All of them said that they didn't think my son was tongue-tied. He continued with swollen tonsils and a speech delay, and I knew something was wrong. I am also a myofunctional therapist and TMJ head and neck physical therapist and knew that my son was posterior tongue-tied but needed someone to diagnose him with it and release it.

I went to Dr. Kotlow and spent the time and effort to go because he was recommended by many of the top lactation consultants and myofunctional therapists. In a matter of one minute, Dr. Kotlow confidently showed me how to diagnose the posterior tongue-tie and successfully released it within ten more minutes.

My son is doing fantastic...he now is talking much much more. I am so grateful that Dr. Kotlow is performing these frenectomies because there are very few dentists or doctors that understand how to diagnose and release these posterior tongue-ties.

Thank you so much for helping me with my son's health because I am very aware of the effects of having a tongue-tie. Now, my son can grow and develop normally.

I am forever grateful for your skill and dedication.

*   *   *

Dr. Kotlow saved my breastfeeding experience with our first child! I happen to be a midwife and had a very difficult month after my daughter was born—first was the pain of breastfeeding by day two, visits with lactation consultants, mastitis, and supplementation due to decreased milk supply. We did get her frenulum clipped, but it did not change the situation. By the end of the month, the pain and struggle were too great, and I was done with breastfeeding. The only thing left to try was lasering with Dr. Kotlow. I called his office, and he invited me in the next day...this was the only thing I had not done and had to do before I quit breastfeeding! By the third day after the procedure (he released both the tongue and lingual frenulums) breastfeeding was no longer a sobbing/agonizing experience. I was incredulous! My daughter didn't even have a severe case of tongue-tie; in fact it was posterior, especially since she had already had it clipped. This experience allowed me to continue breastfeeding and gave me more of an intimate knowledge to take to my clients who have challenges with the same issue.

It's been four years since my daughter was born, and I am still ever so grateful to Dr. Kotlow for his empathy for breastfeeding mothers and for the resources available on his website. (Sharon)

* * *

After almost eight weeks of having every problem under the sun with breastfeeding my son, a lactation consultant finally suggested that he might be tongue-tied. I researched symptoms online, and sure enough, we met every symptom. I contacted my pediatrician so he could recommend someone who could fix the problem who was in network with my insurance; Dr. Kotlow was an out-of-network provider, so his services would not be covered. My pediatrician told me that the surgery was unnecessary and to wait until my child was two to see if he developed a lisp and until then not to worry about it. I told him about breastfeeding problems, and he told me to give my breasts a break for two weeks and pump. His PA gave me the numbers of two ENTs who could possibly take care of the tongue-tie in case I wanted a second opinion. Well, neither ENT could get me in for about six weeks. By then I would have given up breastfeeding due to all the pain I was experiencing.

After thinking about the cost of Dr. Kotlow's services, I decided it would be worth it to pay out of pocket in order to try and make breastfeeding more successful for my baby and me. The office got me in within the week, and I am more than pleased with the experience we had. The doctor was pleasant and in-formative. It turns out my son was severely tongue-tied, and his latch was so much better right after the procedure. For all you mothers out there who have issues breastfeeding and sus-pect tongue-tie, contact this office before you get persuaded by your pediatrician that it is not necessary. I am happy that I went beyond my pediatrician and researched the issue further and found Dr. Kotlow. Why should I have waited two years for a problem such as a lisp to develop? Why should I feel like giving up breastfeeding due to pain and other issues when they could be addressed so it could be a more enjoyable and beneficial experience for my son and me? Dr. Kotlow helped me realize I did this to benefit not only my son but also myself.

* * *

Dr Kotlow saved us! We didn't discover her lip and tongue tie until she was 4 months old. We are just about two weeks out from the revision and I have a COMPLETELY different baby now. She is gaining weight, eating well, no more pain for her or me, colic is gone, spitting up is minimal, no more issues. And she is happy. She smiles all the time. I did a lot of research .He even got me in the next day from when I called, probably because they I was so desperate. It really is amazing the difference. He had a revision at 4 weeks old and wasn't gaining any weight. We are now 15 weeks and over 13lbs!!

Thank you Dr. Larry Kotlow

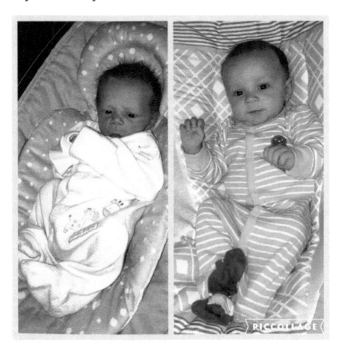

* * *

Owen was born at 36.5 weeks. 6lbs even via C section (presented with arm above his head). Latched on during recovery, 30 minutes or so after he was born. Latched great but very painful. Didn't think anything of it until about 3 days later and I had scabs on my nipples. Was told by the hospital LC that because he was a preemie, he'd be a lazy nurser and just to pump and feed him. I ignored it. Left the hospital at 5lbs 10oz. By 2 weeks, he was at 6lbs 2oz!!!! Yay for gaining. We went in about a week later because Owen started spitting up a ton of milk. They weighed him of course and he was down 2oz. The doctor focused on that and insisted we give him formula. I declined and went home to pump. I asked her to check for ties because at this point I suspected. She grabbed a tongue depressor and looked. Said no ties. She scheduled a weight check for a couple days later. I scheduled an appt with the hospital LC and she didn't feel any ties. Had a weighed feed and was a little under a full feed so wanted us to pump and supplement. Told us that it was because he was a preemie and we'd see a difference soon. We pumped and fed him supplemented a few ounces a day. Went back and he was 6lbs 4oz. However she didn't like the gain and still pushed formula. I told her that with supplementing, he was gaining. She scheduled is for another weight check. At this point, I knew something was up. We went to an oral surgeon who looked with a tongue depressor and said no ties. I was at my wits end with the pumping and feeding so I hired a IBCLC who came to my house. He weighed in at 6lbs 3oz. So she wasn't happy. She had me pumping every 2 hours and supplementing 1oz per feeding. She checked him for ties and said she was pretty sure he had them but couldn't diagnose. At that point, she told me we should see Dr. kotlow in Albany but felt he should be 7lbs first. I didn't like that idea so I called and got an appt for the following Wednesday. She wasn't thrilled that he wasn't 7lbs so I told her I would get him weighed and if he was 6lbs 7oz, I'd take him. And he was! Dr. Kotlow's office said there was no reason to wait. Her reason was that he was so small, he couldn't afford to go longer. We saw a chiropractor the day before the visit and scheduled one for the day after. We took him and was in and out in an hour. Dr. Kotlow told me I wasn't crazy and he had both a tongue and lip tie. We went home with hopes it would all change.

*   *   *

Valerie: Tonight I sat down and shared news with our SLP that my son said 'holiday', 'honeydew', and 'eleven'. "Pepperoni" has been a favorite of his for a while now and he says it... first "me want pepperoni" and this week "I want pepperoni".

SAYS IT! "Pepperoni". Seriously. In weeks past I've said things like"... he's truly exploding with so many words I can't keep up." "His confidence level is very very high right now. He is putting words we've not heard before directly into a sentence." Seriously. In January, JANUARY!! My son was choking on solid foods. Had limited him to a liquid diet, basically. Had been seen by EI for over a year. In that year he gained one 'approximation'. Had seen private SLP's, dentists, lets not even go into our BF experience....JANUARY!! My son had '21 words'. Most of them were 'sound effects' with my husband out of town on business I drove 3 plus hours to Dr Larry Kotlow because I knew we could not wait a day longer. TODAY, just barely over 4 months post-revision my son is speaking in sentences. He has hundreds of words. HUNDREDS! I would pay a hundred PER word, heck his words are priceless! He was straight up three before he said, "love you"Momma's questioning or struggling or guilting - DON'T. I so so so so SO wish I knew my son had a PTT in 2013 NOT 2016.

*   *   *

Rebecca: "I am sitting here enjoying my happy 9 month old son and had a memory of a time when he wasn't so happy. Both of my younger sons were tongue-tied and dealt with GERD as young infants. When my middle child had his tongue-tie corrected at 2 years old we saw not only an improvement in diction and a reduction of GERD symptoms but he also hasn't had any asthma symptoms since having the procedure done. In pediatric patients GERD can irritate the airways and exacerbate reactive airway. I believe having his tongue-tie corrected contributed to his improvement. He is now off of asthma maintenance medications. My youngest had GERD and would cry inconsolably as a young infant; you could hear him refluxing after he ate. He was on medication and was being bottle-fed due to poor weight gain. He is now a happy, fat, healthy 9 month old who loves to nurse.My only regret is that I didn't bring both of my sons to see Dr.Kotlow sooner. Thank you so much!!!!"

REFERENCES

AskMayoExpert. Gastroesophageal reflux in children. 2012.

Bonuck, K, Rau, T, Xu, L. Pediatric Sleep Disorders and Special Educational Need at 8 Years: A Population-Based Cohort Study. *Pediatrics*. 2013;130(4). doi:10.1542/peds.2012-0392d.

Brent, NB. Thrush in the Breastfeeding Dyad: Results of a Survey on Diagnosis and Treatment. *Clinical Pediatrics*. 2001;40(9):503–506. doi:10.1177/000992280104000905.

Buryk, M, Bloom, D, Shope, T. Efficacy of Neonatal Release of Ankyloglossia: A Randomized Trial. *Pediatrics*. 2011;128(2):280–288. doi:10.1542/peds.2011-0077.

Edmonds, J, Miles, SC, Fulbrook, P. Tongue-tie and breastfeeding: a review of the literature. *Breastfeed Rev*. 2011;19(1):19–26.

Flick, RP. Cognitive and Behavioral Outcomes After Early Exposure to Anesthesia. Available at: http://www.vabarnsley.org.uk/pdf/.

Forlenza, GP, Black, NMP, Mcnamara, EG, Sullivan, SE. Ankyloglossia, exclusive breastfeeding, and failure to thrive. *Pediatrics*. 2010;125(6). doi:10.1542/peds.2009-2101.

Gastroesophageal Reflux (GER) and Gastroesophageal Reflux Disease (GERD) in Infants. *Gastroesophageal Reflux (GER) and Gastroesophageal Reflux Disease (GERD) in Infants*. Available at: http://digestive.niddk.nih.gov/ddiseases/pubs/gerdinfant/gerdinfant/. Accessed October 10, 2012.

Hannon, PR, Ehlert-Abler, P, Aberman, S, Williams, R, Carlos, M. A Multidisciplinary Approach to Promoting a Baby Friendly Environment at an Urban University Medical Center. *Journal of Human Lactation*. 1999;15(4):289–296. doi:10.1177/089033449901500403.

Hazelbaker, AK. *Tongue-tie: morphogenesis, impact, assessment and treatment.* Columbus, OH: Aidan and Eva Press; 2010.

Huang, W-JH, Creath, C. The midline diastema: a review of its etiology and treatment. *Pediatric dentistry.* 1995;17(3):171–179.

Jackson, R. Improving breastfeeding outcomes: the impact of tongue-tie. *Community Practitioner.* 2012;85(6).

Jang, S-J, Cha, B-K, Ngan, P, Choi, D-S, Lee, S-K, Jang, I. Relationship between the lingual frenulum and craniofacial morphology in adults. *American Journal of Orthodontics and Dentofacial Orthopedics.* 2011;139(4):361–367. doi:10.1016/j. ajodo.2009.07.017.

Kotlow, L. Diagnosis and treatment of ankyloglossia and tied maxillary fraenum in infants using Er:YaG and 1064 diode lasers. *Eur Arch Paediatr Dent European Archives of Paediatric Dentistry.* 2011;12(2):106–112. doi:10.1007/bf03262789.

Kotlow, L. Infant Reflux and Aerophagia Associated with the Maxillary Lip-tie and Ankyloglossia (Tongue-tie). *Clin Lactn Clinical Lactation.* 2011;2(4):25–29. doi:10.1891/215805311807011467.

Kotlow L. Infant Gastroesophageal Reflux (GER-Benign Infant Acid Reflux) or just Plain Aerophagia? International Journal of Child Health and Nutrition. 2016;5.

Kotlow, L. Oral diagnosis of abnormal frenum attachments in neonates and infants. 2004;10(3):26–28.

Kotlow, L. Oral diagnosis of abnormal frenum attachments in neonates and infants: Evaluation and treatment of the maxillary and lingual frenum using the Erbium:YAG Laser. *Journal of Pediatric Dental Care.* 2004;10(3):11–14.

Kotlow, LA. Diagnosing and Understanding the Maxillary Lip-tie (Superior Labial, the Maxillary Labial Frenum) as it Relates to Breastfeeding. *Journal of Human Lactation*. 2013;29(4):458–464. doi:10.1177/0890334413491325.

Kotlow, LA. The Influence of the Maxillary Frenum on the Development and Pattern of Dental Caries on Anterior Teeth in Breastfeeding Infants: Prevention, Diagnosis, and Treatment. *Journal of Human Lactation*. 2010;26(3):304–308. doi:10.1177/0890334410362520.

Law-Morstatt, L, Judd, DM, Snyder, P, Baier, RJ, Dhanireddy, R. Pacing as a Treatment Technique for Transitional Sucking Patterns. *J Perinatol Journal of Perinatology*. 2003;23(6):483–488. doi:10.1038/sj.jp.7210976.

Livingstone, V. A diagnostic approach to breastfeeding problems. *Canadian J of Ped* . 1990. Available at: http://www.breastfeedingclinic.com/pdf/DiagnosticApproach.pdf.

Maria Stella Amorim Da Costa Zöllner, Jorge, AOC. Candida spp. occurrence in oral cavities of breastfeeding infants and in their mothers' mouths and breasts. *Pesquisa Odontológica Brasileira Pesqui Odontol Bras*. 2003;17(2):151–155. doi:10.1590/s1517-74912003000200010.

Marmet, C, Shell, E, Aldana, S. Assessing infant suck dysfunction: case management. *Journal of Human Lactation*. 2000;16(4):332–336.

Martinelli, R, Marchessen, I, Berretin-Felix, G. Lingual frenulum protocol with scores for infants. *Int J Orofacial Mycology*. 2012;38:104–112.

Meenakshi, S, Jagannathan, N. Assessment of Lingual Frenulum Lengths in Skeletal Malocclusion. *Journal Of Clinical And Diagnostic Research*. 2014;8(3):20–204. doi:10.7860/jcdr/2014/7079.4162.

Mukai, S, Mukai, C, Asaoka, K. Congenital Ankyloglossia with Deviation of the Epiglottis and Larynx: Symptoms and Respiratory Function in Adults. *Annals of Otology, Rhinology & Laryngology.* 1991;100:3–11. doi:10.1177/000348949310200810.

O'Callahan, C, Macary, S, Clemente, S. The effects of office-based frenotomy for anterior and posterior ankyloglossia on breastfeeding. *International Journal of Pediatric Otorhinolaryngology.* 2013;77(5):827–832. doi:10.1016/j.ijporl.2013.02.022.

Palmer, B. Breastfeeding and Frenulums. *Brianpalmerddscom.* Available at: http://www.brianpalmerdds.com/bfeed_frenulums.htm. Accessed March 28, 2016.

Pradhan, S, Yasmin, E, Mehta, A. Management of Posterior Ankyloglossia using the Er,Cr:YSGG Laser. *IJOLD International Journal of Laser Dentistry.* 2012;2:41–46. doi:10.5005/jp-journals-10022-1016.

Sanches, MT. Clinical management of oral disorders in breastfeeding. *Journal of Pediatrics.* 2004;80(5):s155–s162.

Schurr, P. Neonatal mythbusters: evaluating the evidence for and against pharmacologic and nonpharmacologic management of gastroesophageal reflux. *Neonatal Network.* 2012;31:229. Available at: http://nutritioncaremanual.org/index.cfm. Accessed March 28, 2016.

Siegel S. Aerophagia Induced Reflux Associated with Lip and Tongue Tie in Breastfeeding Infants. J Pediatrics. 2016;137(supplement 3).

Siegel S. Aerophagia induced Reflux in breastfeeding Infants with Ankyloglossia and shortened maxillary labial Frenua (Tongue and Lip-Tie) Journal of Clinical Pediatrics 2016;5(1):6-8

Sun, L. Early childhood general anaesthesia exposure and neurocognitive development. *British Journal of Anaesthesia.* 2010;105(Supplement 1):i61–i68. doi:10.1093/bja/aeq302.

Vandenplas Y, et al. Pediatric gastroesophageal reflux clinical practice guidelines: Joint recommendations of the North American Society for Pediatric Gastroenterology, Hepatology, and Nutrition (NASPGHAN) and the European Society for Pediatric Gastroenterology, Hepatology, and Nutrition (ESPGHAN). *Journal of Pediatric Gastroenterology and Nutrition.* 2009;49:498.

Wagoner, C, Rosenkrantz, T. Counseling the breastfeeding mother. *Overview, Mechanics of Breastfeeding, Correct Breastfeeding Techniques.* Available at: http://emedicine.medscape.com/article/979458-overview.

Walls, A, Pierce, M, Wang, H, Steehler, A, Steehler, M, Harley, EH. Parental perception of speech and tongue mobility in three-year olds after neonatal frenotomy. *International Journal of Pediatric Otorhinolaryngology.* 2014;78(1):128–131. doi:10.1016/j.ijporl.2013.11.006.

Watson-Genna, C. *Supporting sucking skills in breastfeeding infants.* Sudbury, MA: Jones and Bartlett Publishers; 2008.

Wiessinger, D, Miller, M. Breastfeeding Difficulties as a Result of Tight Lingual and Labial Frena: A Case Report. *Journal of Human Lactation.* 1995;11(4):313–316. doi:10.1177/089033449501100419.

Winter, HS. Acid reflux (gastroesophageal reflux disease) in children and adolescents. Available at: http://www.uptodate.com/contents/acid-reflux-gastroesophageal-reflux-disease-in-children-and-adolescents-beyond-the-basics. Accessed October 10, 2012.